Schumacher Briefing N

THE ECOLOGY OF HEALTH

Robin Stott

published by Green Books
for The Schumacher Society

First published in 2000
by Green Books Ltd, Foxhole, Dartington, Totnes, Devon TQ9 6EB
www.greenbooks.co.uk greenbooks@gn.apc.org

for The Schumacher Society
The CREATE Centre, Smeaton Road, Bristol BS1 6XN
www.oneworld.org/schumachersoc
schumacher@gn.apc.org

Cover design by Rick Lawrence

Printed by J.W. Arrowsmith Ltd, Bristol, UK

A catalogue record for this publication is available
from the British Library

ISBN 1 870098 80 3

Acknowledgements

Sophie Poklewski Koziell has worked tirelessly in helping me with
both the content and layout of this booklet. I am very grateful to her.
I am also grateful to my family and numerous other friends and
colleagues who have helped me, some spending considerable time
reviewing the text and offering many useful suggestions.
Nevertheless, I alone am responsible for any inaccuracies in the text.

Robin Stott
February 2000

CONTENTS

Foreword

Across the world, the public and politicians are united in their commitment to improve the health of populations. The successes of public health and population control programmes have led to a significant increase in life expectancy in both developed and underdeveloped countries. These successes mean that all these countries are now struggling with the issues of ageing populations and increasing needs for health care. The prominence of the struggle for health care has tended to eclipse the equally important and complementary struggle for health. The need to pursue both in tandem and with vigour is paramount.

In this booklet, Robin Stott brings together the experience and compassion of a clinician caring for individual patients and the strategic approach of a policy analyst who is concerned to influence the determinants of health and disease. He sets out for all health professionals, and for the wider public, the holistic approach that we must take if we are to maintain the improvements in health that have been achieved this century. He emphasises that the advances that we hope for in the 21st century do not depend on further scientific discoveries. He describes the as yet insufficiently recognised relationships between health and our social and physical environment. He then shows how the understanding of these relationships points to the actions that are necessary to improve the physical environment, to reduce inequalities between and within nations, to promote social justice and so to improve our health.

Robin Stott urges us all to recognise our responsibilities for promoting health. He encourages us to have the courage to lend our voices and influence to such a campaign, and to implement policies that go beyond the interests of our patients, to the welfare of citizens everywhere.

Dr June Crown FRCP
Past President of the Faculty of Public Health Medicine

Introduction

Thucydides, on being asked "When will justice come to Athens?", replied: "Justice will come to Athens when those who are not injured are as indignant as those who are."

Looking back at the last few hundred years, there have clearly been enormous developments in health and health care across the world. However, the turn of the millennium offers us all an ideal moment to reflect on the nature and direction of these developments and to ask some pertinent questions.

- Why do so many people across the globe suffer so much ill health?
- Why are health systems in both rich and poor countries groaning under the burden of ill health?
- Why have so many of the improvements in public health been at the expense of the environment?
- Why are so many people turning towards alternative medicines and systems for their health and health care?

We must surely possess the knowledge and resources to create the socially just and environmentally sustainable world that is essential for good health. So what is stopping us?

These questions provided the stimulus for this booklet. I have worked as a hospital doctor in the UK National Health Service (NHS) for 33 years, and my response to these questions is with this experience and from this perspective. Two strands of my work have been particularly important for answering these questions.

Firstly my experience as a clinician, a teacher and in management (as the medical director of a teaching hospital). In my clinical work, my understanding of the need for active listening and empathic communication has gained immeasurably from contact with thousands of patients, their relatives, friends and carers. My considerable management experience has also emphasised for me the importance of working with colleagues from different backgrounds. Furthermore, I have become painfully familiar with the tensions between public and private good, and the inevitable trade-offs that have to be made between quality for one and quality for all. As a teacher, I have enjoyed contact with, and learned much from, students from all branches of the health professions. These students have encouraged me to keep questioning my picture of reality, my way of viewing the world.

Secondly, over these years, the wider implications of health have never been far from my thoughts. I have supported revolutionary health struggles, particularly in Vietnam, sub-Saharan Africa and China, and have come to recognise just how important social injustice is as a barrier to good health. I have also studied Chinese philosophy and Traditional Chinese Medicine (TCM), and worked closely with Zimbabwean traditional healers. Drawing from these experiences, I can appreciate how the social and environmental mind-set of a community determines its thinking on health. Moreover, I realise the profound importance to our health of the way in which we relate to others and to our environment. Working to promote this wider understanding of health in the UK, I have been a member of Medact for 18 years, and, more recently, its chairman. Medact is composed of health profession-als who understand that health is only possible when social and envi-ronmental justice prevails. We research, advocate and campaign on this issue, and Medact further acts as the UK affiliate of two Nobel Peace Prize-winning organisations: International Physicians for Prevention of Nuclear War (IPPNW), and the UK Working Group on Landmines. I am also a member of the UK's Green Party, and over the past twelve years have assisted in the formulation of Green Health, Peace and Security policies. Working within these organisations has enabled me to discuss with colleagues from across the world how best to promote health and deliver health care. I have come to the conclusion that good health can only be realised within the context of true peace and security; and these are dependent on social and environmental justice. The antecedents of both health and security are the same.

These years of immersion have provided helpful insights into health and health care at a local, regional and global level. All of these insights, born of practical experience and illuminated by the thoughtful comments of many friends, colleagues and patients, per-meate this booklet. My core belief is that good health and health care is about a shared vision of what it means to be physically, psychologically, mentally and spiritually fulfilled. It is about:

- recognising the contribution that all of us make to health;
- creating partnerships based on valuing experience as well as scientific knowledge;
- conducting decision-making on an appropriate scale;
- allowing local communities to regain political pre-eminence *vis-à-vis* central and global authorities;
- recreating a sense of meaning and purpose in our everyday lives;
- acknowledging the importance to our health of the water we drink, the air we breathe, the food we eat, the changes in our climate and the amount of radiation we are exposed to;
- acknowledging the health impact of the alcohol we drink, the cigarettes and chemicals we consume, the types of buildings we live in, the distribution of wealth, the size of our communities, the value systems we espouse, and indeed all aspects of our lives; and
- acknowledging, above all, that the health of humanity depends on the health of our planet. We need to be more prudent in the way that we conduct our lives to ensure that the fragile balance between humanity and the planet is not disturbed.

My central message is that the scale at which decisions are made and implemented is of fundamental importance to this wider view of health. Individual and societal health can only be improved if decisions are taken and implemented by people who can:

- relate directly to each other;
- understand the relevance of decisions to their lives;
- determine the size of the constituency which needs to be involved in the decision-making; and therefore
- practice human scale decision-making.

No public health service that I know of is built on this wider view of health, or practices this scale of decision-making. Why does the reality lag so far behind the vision, and how can we bring them closer together? Before we can develop a health and health care system underpinned by the collective action of citizens—citizens who have a large measure of local control and direction over their lives— there are a number of gulfs to bridge:

Between narrow and broad definitions of health. The vast majority of health professionals consider that the 80% of the activities which are undeniably important to our health are none of their concern. This narrow view conflicts with that of the general public, who are bemused by the barriers to their health which grow out of this thinking.

Between the popular understanding of the causes of ill health and our scientific and societal responses to these causes. The popular understanding of health has affinity with the ideas reflected in, for example, Ayurvedic and traditional Chinese medical systems. These emphasise the importance of our whole life experience to our health—a view held by many people but not taken properly into account by health professionals.

Between the wellbeing of the environment and the wellbeing of humans. Much of the social change so important to health over the past 100 years has had adverse environmental consequences. These environmental changes have already begun to undermine any social benefits, and the process is accelerating.

Between a society which pursues wealth in the hope of creating health, rather than health in the hope of creating wealth. The trickle-down theory of development has reached its apotheosis in economic globalisation—a process which has aggravated the divide between rich and poor. Wealth creation which does not occur in a socially and environmentally productive manner necessary to support our wellbeing (through for instance reducing inequalities in income and promoting female education) is not good for health. Health for all is not a beneficiary, but a casualty, of unthinking economic growth.

Between 'power over' and 'power with' leadership. Professionals usually impose decisions, rather than inform decision-making processes.

Between locally determined need and centrally determined actions. When communities are asked what they need from their health system, the answers can be framed as a series of values, which if incorporated can provide the system required. This is only possible in a locally accountable organisation. The health systems in most countries are dominated by centrist thinking and organisation, a process that is getting more difficult to unravel as globalisation takes over.

Between the rhetoric and reality of patient and citizen participation in the control and direction of our lives. There is, as yet, little evidence of a shift in the balance of power from professionals to the wider citizenry.

Even in countries like the UK, which are committed to devolution, the structural changes which will support local decision-making processes are in their infancy. Indeed, countervailing forces are dominant: for instance economic globalisation makes local control and decision-making more difficult and less effective.

Each one of these themes is explored in further detail in the text.

In Chapter 1 (A Holistic View of Health) health is defined broadly. I explain why a broad definition will help reorientate our health services.

In Chapter 2 (A Wider Approach to Health) the necessary societal and environmental preconditions for this broader definition of health are outlined. Issues which have only recently been recognised as important, and those best illustrating how integrated policy can advance health, are explored in detail.

In Chapter 3 (Restoring the Human Scale to Health) the importance of public engagement in transforming health is emphasised, as is how we might enable this. Citizen and patient expectation of our health and health care services is then explored. When these principles are in place, our ideal health service can develop. Using illustrative examples, I argue that this can only be realised in a health system where decisions are taken at a scale determined by local people, who have control over their own destinies, working together.

Finally, in Chapter 4 (The Reorientation of Health and Health Care Systems), practical ways forward are suggested. The evolution and characteristics of organisations which would be both health promoting and able to deliver good health care are explored.

There is a tension threading throughout my text. Much of what I write is critical of the social and organisational systems prevalent in the rich Western world. Yet to change things we have to work within this system. So whilst I offer a radical vision and perspective, I follow the sensible precedents of the Natural Step organisation developed in Scandinavia by Karl-Henrik Robèrt. Change has to be attainable, measurable, made with the support of local people, and evolutionary. It will take many years of hard work to achieve what all of us wish—a healthy humanity living in harmonious balance with each other and with nature—but we can make a start today.

Dr Robin Stott FRCP

Chapter 1

A Holistic View of Health

"To see a world in a grain of sand
And a heaven in a wild flower
Hold infinity in the palm of your hand
And eternity in an hour."
William Blake

From a narrow to a holistic view of health
There is a Sufi parable of five blind men who were asked to feel, and describe, an elephant. The first, touching the elephant's tail, said "The elephant is like a rope." "Rubbish," said the second, after touching its leg, "the elephant is just like a tree trunk." "No," said the third, stroking the elephant's side, "it's like a great wall covered in leather." After touching the ears, the fourth said, "You are all wrong; it's like a leathery bird with huge wings." Finally the fifth, feeling the trunk, said "No—it's like a serpent." Knowing only the parts, and blind to the whole, these sincere men came to very different, and inaccurate, conclusions about the elephant. Health is an equally elusive concept, and whilst many have tried to describe parts of it, few have captured the totality.

The measures of health customarily used by professionals perpetuate confusion over what we mean by health. Measures such as life expectancy and infant mortality are assumed to reflect the activities of the health service, but fail to do so. *Per capita* expenditure on 'health' reflects the amount we spend on health care, but is of little relevance to health. The same is true for the number of contacts between health professionals and patients, bed days in hospital, operations done and waiting lists, all of which are measures of the quantity of health *care*. Each of these measures reflect only part of the 'elephant of health', and are no measure of the whole. This is not surprising, as 80% of our health is determined by policies and activities outside the conventional health sector, for instance transport and housing policy, farming practice and the level of violence in society. These wider policies do not get appropriate credit in the current measurements of health.

The partial perspective that the existing measurements of health give us explains the anomaly of modern societies, which should (according to official measurements) be feeling better, but are actually (using more relevant indicators) feeling worse. Aaron Wildasky ascribed this paradoxical situation to what he called the 'political pathology of health', in which medical care (what in terms of the Sufi parable we might call 'the tail of health'), is equated to the whole elephant of health. Our confusion about the meaning of health also leads to the problem of trying to measure 'progress' in health and health care. Whether health is improving or deteriorating depends on which part of the elephant we look at.

Health and health care: improving or deteriorating?
On one hand our health has never seemed better, and our health care never more all-embracing. International statistics show that even in many underprivileged areas of the world, life expectancy is increasing, infant mortality decreasing, and immunisation rates are improving.[1] In the rich North, diagnostic and therapeutic possibilities unimaginable only a few years ago are now commonplace. For instance, when I started practice in 1966 there were no endoscopies, CAT (computerised axial tomography) scans or ultrasound; external cardiac massage was only just being introduced; and most of today's commonly used drugs had not been developed. The speed of change is bewildering. The perceived power of 'scientific medicine' has been bolstered by these changes, which have contributed to the wildly optimistic expectations of curative medicine which so many of us have. Moreover, the sequencing of the human genome, due to be completed by 2002, is likely to unleash a whole spectrum of revolutionary health technologies.[2]

On the other hand, when different areas of health are examined, serious problems come to light. For instance, the disparity in wealth both between and within nations promotes much ill health.[3] Malnutrition affects one billion of our global population, and simple dietary diseases such as iron and iodine deficiency are rampant,[4] with women bearing the brunt of all these problems. The global malaria situation is becoming worse: some 1.5–2.7 million people die of this disease every year, mainly in tropical Africa. Heart disease is the major killer of the two billion members of the affluent classes, and is more common in those who feel a lack of engagement in their lives and work.[5] Many cancers have clear environmental associations—such as exposure to chemicals and radiation.[6] HIV infection, which is devastating sub-Saharan Africa, now afflicts 33 million people.[7] Tuberculosis causes a quarter of all preventable adult deaths, and 95% of the 8 million new cases each year are in the poorer countries.[8] Violence is pandemic, with the 20th century witnessing genocide, wars and criminal and domestic violence of an unprecedented intensity. Persistent organic pollutants (POPs)—fat soluble, long-lasting byproducts of 20th century manufacturing—not only threaten to undermine human fertility, but also to poison present and future generations. These social and environmental problems also adversely affect our mental health.[9] The markers of positive mental health—our capacity to be at peace with ourselves, to enjoy intimate relationships, to have a sense of purpose and to feel the enchantment of living[10]—are stunted by our present circumstances. Indeed our mental health is so threatened that psychotropic drugs are expected to be the most commonly prescribed drugs in the new century. Compounding all this, our physical environment, the ultimate source of our wellbeing, is continuously being assailed from all sides.

Meanwhile, health care systems in the richest countries groan under the financial burden of ill health. Clinicians in my hospital 'doing their rounds' frequently treat people lying on trolleys in the Accident and Emergency Department, and people die of heart disease whilst awaiting treatment. In poor countries, health care systems are already an acknowledged disaster area. In most hospitals in Africa even the most basic facilities, such as water or power, are only intermittently available. All over the world patients complain about both too much and too little treatment, and believe that technology and professionalism sometimes displace care and compassion. Meanwhile, countless patients seek help not from the 'scientific' medicines, but from the many traditional systems of health care.

The example of the UK
The manner in which a society understands health ultimately shapes health policy. Therefore confusions about definitions of health not only make measurement difficult, but also disrupt the evolution of the health service. This has happened in the UK: in 1949, when the

National Health Service (NHS), a public service, was formed, its founder—Aneurin Bevan—believed that health care delivered free at the point of use would improve the overall health of the public. He imagined that through using health care facilities, the public would all become so healthy that their reliance on the health service would gradually reduce. However, this was not to be. He did not fully appreciate how little the 'health service' contributes to overall health. Given our present understanding of the determinants of good health, we can now see that Bevan's aspirations could never be realised. The misconceptions on which the NHS was founded proved to be an insurmountable obstacle. Moreover, in the intervening years, the gulf between improving our health and the delivery of 'health care' has become ever more pronounced. The noble ideal of the 'National Health Service' has been replaced by the reality of a 'National Disease Service'.

The cost of the disease service has escalated dramatically, partly because of the introduction of costly new technologies and also because we have not invested sufficiently in the social and environmental factors that underpin true health. In 1949 'the health service' consumed 3% of GDP. Now delivering health care in the UK currently costs around £40 billion a year—6% of a much larger GDP. Today, most UK health professionals at least recognise the pre-eminent importance of wider social, environmental and educational policy in improving health.[11,12] Those working in health care recognise that £40 billion has little impact on the overall health of the nation. However, where this money is spent well, the benefits in terms of comfort, care and cure are immense, and this is the raison d'être of most health care workers.

What many health professionals choose to ignore is the need for change in the framework of our thinking about health. If we wish to move from our present 'disease service' to a true 'health service', we must avoid the pitfalls that snared the architects of not only the UK health service, but also those of nearly every other country worldwide. We need policy initiatives which promote both health and health care. This is no more than a return to traditional medical systems, in which the delivery of health and health care are so closely entwined as to be indistinguishable. The reality of our present health system is far from this. Part of the solution here proposed is to combine the delivery of health and health care in a coherent framework.

The need for a wider definition of health

To accomplish this, to build truly healthy societies, we must move to a wider definition of health. We must take each part of the definition, each part of the elephant of health, and show how it is integrated to create the whole animal. This will provide us with a framework within which we can develop appropriate policies. Only then will we be able to infuse our present health systems with the inspiration and energy needed to make the necessary changes.

I have described health as a state in which individuals are physically, psychologically, mentally and spiritually fulfilled, and so can lead fulfilling lives both now and in the future (Box 1). This state is best realised when, treasuring the diversity and beauty of our planet and of each other, people achieve control over their lives. It demands an equitable distribution of power and resources both within and between societies. A fulfilling life can only be sustained by preserving the integrity of our environment. Health is a collective value. One person's health should not, and ultimately cannot, be maintained at the expense of another's, nor through the excessive use of natural resources.

The next chapter explores the determinants of health, and shows how integrating each of these into a coherent whole will allow us to create a society in which good health will flourish.

Box 1: A fulfilling life

A fulfilling life is described by individuals who have benefited from all of Maslow's well-known categories of need:

- the basic physiological needs of air, water, food and sex;
- the needs for safety and security, adequate shelter, safe circumstances and fulfilling employment;
- the need for love and belonging to friends, family and community;
- the need for self-esteem through respect for others and oneself; and
- the need for a sense of purpose, and a sense of the joy of living.

These needs are both hierarchical and interrelated. Without air, water and food, safety and security become meaningless. Similarly, having a sense of joy in life and a sense of purpose are made extremely difficult if other levels of need are not in place. But people's capacity to experience love and self-esteem, for instance, can thread through each of the other levels.

Chapter 2
A Wider Approach to Health

"There is no psychological truth unless it be particular, but on the other hand there is no art unless it be general. The whole problem lies in just that—how to express the general by the particular—how to make the general express the particular." André Gide

I do not want to mar the arrival of the new millennium by crafting too rigid a definition of health. The descriptions I have used enable us to gain a clear understanding of the factors that contribute to our health. They imply that our collective and individual health depends on the following:

- the social circumstances in which we live (our social arrangements);
- our relationships with our fellow beings (our community relations); and
- the way we interact with our built environment, with nature and thus with the planet (our environmental relations).

Much of this knowledge is not new, and doctors in previous centuries were aware of these general prescriptions for health. For instance in the UK Public Health Act of 1848, clean air and water, nourishing, unadulterated food and weatherproof, well-insulated houses were identified as being important for health. Over the years, the relative importance attached to these factors has changed, and we have added others, such as effective transport, to the list. We also have a clearer idea of the role of the environment in supporting our health.

What is new in the public health debate is the emphasis on the less visible aspects of our social arrangements, such as relative poverty, powerlessness, and loss of community, which are now known to be important to our health. Moreover, there is a new realisation that in trying to build healthy societies, environmental problems have been created which endanger our own health and the health of the planet. We in the rich North have built a society in which we have clean water, good housing, plenty of food but at the cost of polluting our air, our land and our rivers. Meanwhile in the South, IMF and World Bank attempts to reduce poverty through economic structural adjustment programmes have not only failed to produce social benefit but have also often lead to environmental degradation. We have not fully appreciated that the waxing of one aspect of health can lead to the waning of another. We have forgotten the wisdom of many pre-industrial societies, which recognised that to live in harmony with nature is to ensure sustained good health.

What is also new to health discussions is the importance of learning from the past, as I have recognised in my conversations with health professionals interested in complementary medicine. If we learn from the old ways of delivering health, such as the traditional health systems of China (see Box 2) and India, we can receive new health benefits. These philosophies emphasise the importance of identity of the human with the natural environment, as well as stressing the importance of mind, body and spirit in health. They also emphasise the necessity of involving people in their health care.

We must recognise the potential health problems in store if we transgress the basic principles of interdependence between humans and nature. The lessons of history are there for all to see: Easter Island, the cities of the Euphrates valley, and the extraordinary Mogul capital of Fatipur Sikri were all abandoned because their people failed to live in harmony with their environment. If we do not want to follow these once great civilisations into oblivion, we must heed the warning signs that they no doubt ignored. Today's warning signs are only too clear: fractured, violent and impoverished communities; global warming; soil erosion; polluted and dwindling fresh water supplies; and extinction of species.

In what follows, I categorise the basic antecedents of health. Then I focus on some of the less well recognised causes of ill health, as well as the interrelationships between the various individual causes. I stress that in health policy there is no such thing as a single issue, everything is interrelated—so in addressing one problem it is important not to create another.

**Box 2: Traditional Chinese Medicine—
incorporating environmental and social factors into health**

TCM has always recognised the relationships between the physical and social environment and health. From my personal experience and training in TCM, and from discussion with many colleagues and patients, I have learnt the following lessons from this ancient medical system and the many others that still persist throughout the world.

Firstly, TCM taught me to understand—more clearly than any of my conventional medical practice—the importance of our physical and social environment to our health. Preventative medicine has to deal with social and environmental concerns, such as fostering appropriate relationships within our communities, housing, pollution and education, as well as the narrower health targets advocated by our Departments of Health. To put this in the context of our present analysis, TCM recognises that health depends on social capital and environmental balance, and that both these are best realised through the direct interaction of individuals with each other and with their environment—interactions facilitated where necessary by trusted health workers.

TCM also clarified for me the importance of environmental and lifestyle changes in the curing of disease. The essence of what I learned is that the TCM world-view bridges the gulfs outlined in the Introduction. It is the medicine of humanity and scale, where health professionals and patients understand health care and health in a considered and integrated way, and reflect human rights and responsibilities with compassion.

Another aspect of TCM is the insight it gives us into the wisdom of our world's oldest surviving culture. The intuitive understanding that TCM offers on the fundamental physical and social structures of society are remarkably similar to many of the insights that we are getting both from modern management theory and from modern physics.[13]

Finally, TCM reminds us Western doctors of the need to take into account the whole person in our medical practice, and of our place as individuals embedded in an environment upon which we depend for our continued existence.

Our social environment

Our social environment, within which I include the political and economic systems that regulate our lives, is built on the basis of interactions between people at a series of levels in society. There are a number of desirable characteristics arising from these social interactions, which cumulatively contribute to the public health. They include the following:

Employment—rewarding and rewarded contributions to society

Maximising the number of people engaged in rewarding, rewarded and useful work is a public health issue. Long term unemployment exacerbates poverty, isolation, depression and powerlessness, and can have a serious effect on health, especially mental health. Formal full-time employment is no longer the norm in many societies as work patterns evolve into many forms, from full-time and part-time employment to voluntary work in the community. Schemes such as Local Economy Trading Schemes (LETS) and Time Dollars can revolutionise local work patterns, with substantial public health gain (see Box 3). There is also great potential for employment in a sustainable, health-promoting economy, such as in organic farming, public transport, caring for the sick, and renewable energy.

Empowerment

The degree of democracy and local participation in decision-making is increasingly seen as a key component to health. The social and environmental arrangements for health can only be realised when people are agents, not objects, of change. A healthy society would aim for an equitable distribution of power and a high degree of local participation in decision-making, so that individuals feel that they have a say in, and an appropriate degree of control over, their lives. As well as formal democratic participation, this would mean that the many methods of engaging the public with a view to developing a habit of citizenship should be deployed.

The role of women

Since women have key roles in all societies with respect to basic living conditions, representation of women is particularly important in improving health status. Yet women remain largely under-represented at most levels of government, especially in ministerial and other executive bodies. A more equal representation of women in

Box 3: LETS and Time Dollars

Time Dollars (TDs)—sometimes called Time Money—are a complementary currency that credit the time people spend helping each other. Participants earn credits for doing jobs—an hour of your time entitles you to an hour of someone else's time. Credits are deposited centrally in a 'time bank' and withdrawn when participants need help themselves. TDs can fuel patient support groups, telephone services, bereavement counselling and self-help groups. It makes health a way of living and sharing and acknowledges that active communities are healthy communities.

In the US, TDs have transformed health service users from consumers into producers. Some health insurers encourage older people to pay a quarter of their insurance charge in TDs because they keep older people healthy and in their own homes. In Japan, a version of TDs is used by the Sawayaka Welfare Institute (SWI).[14] They run a scheme in which people caring for the elderly are paid in a special currency called Caring Relationship Tickets. Each ticket represents an hour of service. Non-profit organisations issue the tickets and the people providing the services lodge them in a health care time savings account from which they can draw if ever they need care themselves. Most people assign their credits to their parents. It is predicted that in Japan this system will soon cover 30-50% of the cost of caring for the elderly.

LETS schemes use specialised local currencies to get local economies moving again. This means that people can exchange goods and services even when the local community has run out of conventional cash. It also allows people who may not have full employment to participate in the local economy. In return for doing work for someone else on the scheme, participants earn local currency. They can use this to pay other participants to do something that they cannot do themselves, or might not have the money to pay for. Both LETS and the different forms of Time Money give people the opportunity to be involved in rewarding—and rewarded—employment, some of which is directly related to health-enhancing activities. Moreover, for the long-term unemployed it can help to counter isolation, depression and poverty, as well as rebuilding and establishing community relationships and economies.

politics and decision-making positions would help to redefine political priorities, place new items on the political agenda, and provide new perspectives on mainstream political issues.

Reducing poverty

Poverty is undoubtedly a public health issue. Ultimately, only an equitable distribution of wealth—sufficient to eliminate absolute poverty—can reverse relative poverty and so enable people to live in more healthy and balanced communities.

Social inclusion

A healthy society is one in which there is easy and equitable access to services, including family planning, pre-school childcare, education, training, health care and affordable housing.

Food production, distribution and diet

Health-enhancing and environmentally sensitive food production is another key to good health. Additionally, reducing the distance between farm and fork, and increasing choice and access to healthy food across society, are crucial.

Minimal violence and crime

A social environment where people can live without fear of violence against either themselves or their property is essential to good health. A community in which there is a high level of trust between members is one in which crime and violence is much reduced. War is one of the world's most serious threats to health. For every combatant killed in war, one non-combatant is also killed directly, 14-15 civilians lose their lives from loss of shelter, food, and water or epidemics—and several times these numbers are physically or psychologically wounded.[15] Wars also hinder or destroy health programmes.

Community support

People living in communities characterised by social fragmentation are likely to have increased rates of suicide. Social networks, such as self-help groups and community centres, help to create trusting communities and to prevent alienation and provide support at all levels. A range of local cultural and community activities, to which people are connected and with which they are engaged, are integral to promoting health.

The assets that emerge from these social arrangements and community relations can be described as 'Social Capital' (here the term is used more widely than as a measure of trust within a community). We already have, or can easily develop, measures for each of the individual assets, which can be aggregated to give a measure of social capital. Thus social capital is an indicator of the extent to which the social foundation of a society promotes health.

In order to create the strong vibrant communities that are the basis of a healthy society, we need to invest resources and effort in building each of the above assets. None can be built without the direct interaction of people with each other. Nor, given the enormous disparities of wealth and opportunity that exist worldwide, can the investment be made without a transfer of resources from the rich to the poor. This transfer will lead to a 'convergence' of resources. Convergence describes the move to reduce social inequalities, and can be used as a shorthand description of the move towards social justice. Convergence, so defined, can only be accomplished through the direct interaction of people with each other. This interaction should be illuminated by the principle of 'Do as you would be done by'.

No discussion of social arrangements is complete without reference to population control. Although this is of crucial importance, reducing and sustainable populations can only be secured through the construction of the socially supportive environment that is essential to health. All the evidence that is presently available suggests that the evolution of a globally supportable population will be achieved in concert with a healthy society.

Our physical environment
Our physical environment supports our health in four broad ways:

- as a source of energy and materials;
- as a sink for pollution and other waste;
- as a service for water, nutrients and carbon recycling; and
- as a space for living, working and aesthetics.

Thus the most important determinants of a health-promoting physical environment are:

A continuing supply of clean water and clear air

Today 20% of the global population lack access to an adequate supply of safe drinking water, and an estimated 50% lack a sanitary means of excreta disposal. Yet even without satisfying these basic health needs for a great many people, our global demand for water for domestic, agricultural and industrial purposes is ever-increasing; the total water demand increased by six times between 1900 and 1990, more than double the rate of population growth for the same period. Not surprisingly, water scarcity today is increasingly threatening human health. Freshwater resources are also vulnerable, not only through overexploitation, but also as a result of poor management and ecological degradation. Untreated sewage, industrial waste and agricultural run-off containing herbicides and pesticides are all constantly discharged into water courses. All these have serious implications for health, now and in the future.

Sufficient unpolluted soil

Unpolluted soil is a prerequisite for health. Increasingly the quality (through pollution by POPs, heavy metals and radioactive chemicals) and quantity (through topsoil erosion) of the soil is being undermined, with implications for food production and fresh water supplies.

The maintenance of a stable atmosphere

There has been mounting evidence that our world is warming, and it has now been confirmed that these changes are due to human activities. The Intergovernmental Panel on Climate Change has forecast a 1°–3.5°C increase in average global temperature by 2100. The potential impact of global climate change on human health includes an increase in the frequency of flooding, heatwaves and episodes of air pollution, as well as a change in the distribution and seasonality of diseases.

An environment in which the risk of accidents is minimised

Accidents are a major cause of demands on the health care system, whether at the primary health care or hospital level. On average, in the industrialised countries (and also in many developing countries) one hospital bed in ten is occupied by an accident victim. And in regions of the Americas, accidents are among the five leading causes of death. The health consequences are significant, and greatly underestimated by the public and even by top-level decision-makers. Traffic accidents, in particular, are a major cause of severe injuries in most countries (see

Box 4). Preventing accidents in the home, work, school and community, plays an important part in promoting public health.

Facilities for encouraging active life styles

The present affluent consumer societies of the 'Rich North' militate against physical exercise, and these societies have justly been called obesogenic societies. An obesogenic society provides fertile soil for the evolution of many of the diseases of Western civilisation. Efforts to promote activity and exercise as a normal part of daily life are important ways of mitigating the diseases so prevalent in obesogenic societies (see Box 7).

Adequate housing

Housing should be affordable and also appropriately insulated against the extremes of temperature and noise. Good housing minimises disease and injury, and contributes much to physical, mental and social wellbeing.

Environmental sustainability

Crucially, all of the above requirements must be developed within the limits of environmental sustainability. This will ensure that any changes made are long-lasting and not counterproductive.

Box 4: Reducing traffic accidents in Denmark

In the early 1970s, Denmark had the highest rate of child mortality from traffic accidents in Western Europe. A pilot project was started in Odense, with an ongoing budget of approximately $150,000 a year. Forty-five schools participated in an exercise carried out with accident specialists, planning officials, the police, hospitals and road authorities to identify the specific road dangers that needed to be addressed. As a result, a network of traffic-free foot and bicycle paths was created, as well as a parallel policy of traffic speed reduction, road narrowing and traffic islands. Following the success of the pilot study, the Danish "Safe Routes to Schools" Programme has been implemented in 65 out of 185 proposed localities. By creating networks of cycling and walking routes, changing street design, and installing traffic-calming and traffic-reduction measures in key areas, the number of accidents has fallen by 85%.[16] This is one example of how changing the physical environment can prevent accidents.

Within this list of social and environmental needs, there are many whose impact on health is obvious and easy to understand, such as poor housing, polluted water, inadequate food and absolute poverty. In what follows, we focus on aspects of the social and physical environment that are less visible, and are on the fringes of discussions about health, but are increasingly recognised as important to health.

Poverty and its impact on health

Poverty is a public health issue. It is defined as limited purchasing power and limited access to resources, and in both poor and rich societies it is a sensitive indicator of health. The links between poverty and health are explained through financial, psychological and behavioural factors:

- Financial: income provides the means of obtaining the fundamental prerequisites of life, such as shelter, food, warmth and the ability to participate in society.
- Psychological: living with limited access to resources creates stress, limits choices and reduces ability to solve problems. All these are associated with poor health.
- Behavioural: poverty may lead to health-damaging behaviour. Poor people may degrade their environment out of necessity, whereas rich people more often do so out of greed. Poor people are more prone to individually damaging activities, such as smoking and alcohol abuse.

The health implications of absolute poverty are not in doubt. In 1999, around 1.3 billion people worldwide lived on less than $1 per day, the arbitrary definition of absolute poverty (the dollar is set at 1985 levels). These people have little access to clean water or food and usually have little education. 70% of both the malnourished and illiterate are female, and many of them are children—malnutrition affects one third of the world's children. The prevalence of deficiency and infectious diseases for which there are simple and inexpensive treatments is very high.[17] The contrast between the 'least developed countries', where more than 20% of children die before they reach the age of 5, and typical 'developed countries', where less than 1% of children will do so, indicates that we are far from doing as well as we would like, or in fact could.

However, what is now equally clear is the role of *relative* poverty as a marker of poor health. The health implications of relative poverty were rediscovered in Britain and in the USA in the 1960s.[18, 19] A boy of professional or managerial parents has a life expectancy five years greater than one born to parents in partly skilled or unskilled occupations,[20] and morbidity is also higher in poor children. In London the chances of dying before 75 years of age is almost twice as high in the deprived, impoverished boroughs as compared with the affluent ones. Measuring changes in absolute and relative poverty can therefore be used as surrogate markers for improving health.

Powerlessness and its impact on health

Powerlessness is also a public health issue. There is an increased prevalence of many illnesses among those who feel powerless to control their lives. One of the clearest studies of this was the health survey of over 7,000 UK civil servants.[21] Those in lower employment grades had more heart disease that was not accounted for by the usual risk factors. What mattered to their health was the level of control that these civil servants had over their working lives. Poor control increased workers' stress levels, causing changes in the body's metabolism, and predisposed them to heart disease. Some of the increase in mortality in lower socio-economic groups is accounted for by this feeling of lack of control.

It follows that major health benefits are to be gained by increasing the degree of control that individuals have both inside and outside the work place. Within the workplace, an environmental and social impact assessment (ESIA—see Box 11) is a way of measuring the extent of people's participation in the affairs of their organisation, and the quality and sustainability of the working environment.

The results of the assessments can be used for measuring and then improving health. ESIAs can be used at any level of society, but can only be effective as tools for health improvement when the means and structures are available for citizens to participate in the organisation of their societies (and so to have a greater degree of control over their destinies). New methods of democratic participation are being developed, such as planning for real exercises, Citizens' Juries, citizens' panels, and focus groups. Citizens' Juries have already been used by health authorities to address health policy questions (see Box 5). There are also many other innovative ways of engaging the public that need to be further assessed.

Powerlessness and Globalisation

Given that our definition of public health is one of healthy people living in environmentally sustainable circumstances, the impact of economic globalisation (see Box 6) can only cause a deterioration in health. Indeed, economic growth that has not been used for improving social and environmental arrangements is the source of many of our health problems. Although many industrialised nations now recognise that health is good for the economy, none have yet fully appreciated how bad the economy might be for health. The reality is that the unrestrained pursuit of wealth does not necessarily improve health.

One potent marker of the impact of globalisation is the increasing gap between the rich and the poor. In 1970, the richest 20% of humanity had roughly 30 times more income than the poorest 20%. Today, the richest fifth receive more than 60 times as much as the poorest fifth does. The UK is one country where this widening gap is particularly apparent. For instance, between 1979 and 1995, average incomes grew by about 40%. For the richest tenth of the population, growth was 60-68%, but for the poorest tenth it was only 10% (before housing costs) or a fall of 8% (after them).[22] The overall income inequality in the UK was greater in the mid-1990s than at any time since the late 1940s. We know that this further impoverishment of the poor is a marker of deteriorating health.

An antidote to globalisation, and the best prescription for health, is the reconstruction of local economies through the democratic inclusion of all people. To facilitate the transition of global to local economies, environmental and social impact assessments should be given priority over economic considerations in any government or industrial policy. In addition, human and environmentally sensitive indicators should be used as markers of a society's wealth.[23] To design new systems that will nurture our health and deliver effective health care, we must refuse to be cowed by the prevailing world view implanted in our minds of a single world dominated by insatiable market forces. We need to adopt new approaches that should not conform to the globalisation and growth mantra.

Trust within a community, and health

Cohesive communities in which there is a high level of trust between members are healthy communities. This intuitive feeling is supported

Box 5: Citizens' Juries and health policy

Citizens' Juries (CJs) are a new model for public involvement in decision-making. They involve the public in their capacity as ordinary citizens, and they aim to combine information, time, scrutiny, deliberation and independence in addressing questions of national or local importance.

A model for CJs in the UK, based on similar models from the USA and Germany, has been developed by the Institute of Public Policy Research. In this model, 12-16 jurors, broadly representative of their community, are recruited and are asked to address an important question about policy, or planning, over four days. Jurors scrutinise the information given to them, cross-examine witnesses, discuss and deliberate. Their conclusions are then compiled in a report. The commissioning authority is required to publicise the jury and its findings, to respond within a set time and either to follow its recommendations, or explain publicly why it will not.

In 1996 in the UK, a range of health authorities commissioned a pilot series of CJs. Questions of rationing were high on the health policy agenda, and as unelected bodies, health authorities were facing a crisis of legitimacy as they were obliged to take increasingly controversial decisions about setting priorities and allocating resources. Such issues could not be tackled by clinicians and managers alone, but needed input from the wider public. CJs were convened to address single policy issues such as whether the public should be involved in setting priorities for rationing health care, and how citizens should pay for health care in the future.

At around £16-20,000 for a four-day jury, CJs are a relatively time-consuming and costly exercise compared to opinion polls, public meetings or focus groups. But evidence suggests that they are better at tackling complex questions and difficult choices than other models. Moreover, it was clear from the pilot studies that ordinary citizens are willing to get involved in decision-making processes. The results of the CJs also showed that the public have strong and consistent views about the kind of health service that they want for themselves and their families.

by the work of Syme and Putnam in their work with American and Italian communities.[24,25] Social networks, reflected by the range of local cultural and community activities that people are engaged in, are indicators of a supportive community. These networks are important in the building of trust, and help to increase the sense of community and to counter alienation. They can also provide support for those who, for instance, drink to excess or smoke cigarettes. Nevertheless, however cohesive a community is, breakdowns in communication will occur. Resolving these through mediation is essential to nourishing trust. There are many groups who can give helpful advice about mediation, and from whose experiences we should learn.

Access to healthy foods and exercise—its impact on health
A poor diet is a public health issue. Diet is dependent on the type of food available, food production and distribution. Access to a balanced diet, with appropriate amounts of carbohydrate, protein and fat, trace elements and vitamins, is vital for life. Billions of people in the developing world have an inadequate supply of one or more of these basic necessities. This is usually because the poor have no means of providing themselves with a stable diet. An estimated 58% of pregnant women in developing countries are anaemic, with the result that their infants are more likely to be born with low birth weight and depleted iron stores. Worldwide, 1.3 billion people suffer from starvation.

On the other hand, it is the amount of foods eaten, and lack of relationship between food and exercise, which give rise to one of today's principal neglected public health problems—obesity. The prevalence of obesity in adults is 10%–25% in most countries of Western Europe, 20%–25% in some countries in the Americas, up to 40% in some countries in Eastern Europe, and more than 50% in some countries in the Western Pacific. It is a global problem—both developed and developing countries are affected—and is increasing worldwide at an alarming rate. Obesity is a significant risk factor for a range of serious non-communicable diseases, accidents, and other serious health problems. It has been suggested that of the more than 10 million cases of cancer that occurred in 1996, an estimated 30-40% are preventable by feasible, appropriate diets, and by physical activity and maintenance of appropriate body weight. With obesity rates doubling every 5-10 years in many parts of the world, the financial strain on health systems is evident. In the United States it has been estimated to contribute to 8% of all illness costs (around £40 billion a year).

What causes obesity? A recent shift in thought has moved away from counting calories to the idea of the 'obesogenic environment'—one that encourages obesity. This includes motorised transport, mechanised equipment, and the fact that few people's work

Box 6: Globalisation and health—a new problem

The world economy has changed its nature-since the early 1970s. It has become highly unstable, and has favoured the rich over the poor. A number of changes have taken place which help explain why this has happened:

- On 15th August 1971, President Nixon took the USA off the gold standard, thereby removing the last fixed link between paper money and real goods. In the 1990s, with the escalation of futures, spots and derivatives, only about 10% of money is supported by tangible goods.
- Trade has been liberalised, with the free movement of capital promoted by the lifting of exchange controls, and now enshrined in World Trade Organisation policies.
- This lack of regulation and of border controls enables financial markets to merge into single unregulated electronic trading systems prone to speculative excess.
- The faceless traders running this system move 2 trillion dollars around the world every day.
- The transnational institutions that are the main beneficiaries of the money, lack any kind of accountability to either the public or the environment.

David Korten's[25] analysis of the impact of this globalisation is:

- it depletes natural capital by stripping forests and dumping hazardous wastes on once productive land;
- it depletes human capital by maintaining substandard working conditions in many parts of the world;
- it depletes social capital by driving down wages, uprooting industries and moving them to cheaper locations; and
- it depletes institutional capital by undermining the necessary function and credibility of local democratic governance.

This has lead to a situation where a large proportion of the world's population has lost the means to provide for itself, and has become dependent on a single, highly volatile economic system that has no apparent use for a growing proportion of the people. This removal of large numbers of people from any participation in the global economy deepens the sense of powerlessness that is now such a pervasive feature of our societies.

involves physical activity (only 20% of men and 10% of women are employed in active occupations in the UK). For many, leisure time pursuits are dominated by television viewing—which has been identified in the USA as the most important determinant of childhood and adolescent obesity.

Health professionals can play a strong role in encouraging physical exercise (see Box 7). For instance, more counselling by doctors on this subject increased activity levels amongst sedentary adults in Australia and New Zealand. However this is only part of the solution. Community infrastructure is seen to be an important determinant of encouraging daily physical activity. In the United States 1% of all trips are by bicycle (as compared with 30% in the Netherlands) and 9% are by walking (as compared with 18% in the Netherlands). The Netherlands has community infrastructure and cultural norms that supports physical activity. These are just some of the factors needed to reverse the move towards an 'obesogenic society'.

Food quality also has an impact on health. Food scares, such as bovine spongiform encephalopathy (BSE) in the UK and dioxins in animal feed in Belgium, highlight the problems with intensive livestock raising and food-chain issues. Battery farming and other high intensity practices necessitate the extensive use of antibiotics in feeds—one example of how food production methods threaten human health. Health professionals encourage the intake of fruit and vegetables to promote a healthy diet, but many of these foods are grown and stored with excessive use of agrochemicals. This has serious implications for food quality. Carrots are sprayed with an average of four insecticides, three herbicides and two fungicides. Lettuces are sprayed up to 15 times and an estimated 30% of residue from spraying bananas ends up in the fruit.[26] A UK government survey in 1997 found evidence of 32 different agrochemicals leaving detectable traces in apples. A rapid move to organic farming would reduce many of these problems.

The distribution of food also has health consequences. Food grown and sold locally supports the local economy. In many poor countries, local food production is one of the few ways in which people can defend their local economies from the ravages of economic globalisation. The distance that food travels between production and consumption (food miles) also has significant

Box 7: Exercise prescription schemes

Exercise prescription schemes have been widely introduced in many areas of the UK. One such GP Exercise Referral Scheme has been running since 1993 in Devon, UK.[27] The project was set up as a partnership between the local council, local health authority and local GPs.

The scheme works in the following way. Health professionals issue those patients who they think would benefit from exercise with a referral card. The patients then visit the local leisure centre, which (through council financial support) offers a free assessment and personalised exercise training at a reduced cost. After three months people are offered a reassessment, and recommended to visit their GP again to discuss their health.

At first, GPs generally referred those patients who were unfit or obese, but soon recognised that the scheme gave significant benefits to people with psychological disorders, particularly depression and anxiety. The scheme was later extended to include a special programme for people with arthritis and back pain.

So far, over 2000 people have taken part in this scheme. As a result of the programme, fitness levels and sense of wellbeing are generally improved: 64% showed a reduction in blood pressure, 44% of patients lost weight and 34% increased their weight. Patients report that they are eating a more healthy diet, and drinking and smoking are reduced. Moreover, at the end of their exercise programme a third of patients took up a monthly membership with the leisure centre, and over half continued to drop in casually. As well as creating an 'exercise culture' in the town, a forum for social interaction has developed which is has proved invaluable for many people who were previously socially isolated.

environmental consequences. For instance, millions of bananas from Honduras and kiwi fruit from New Zealand now travel further than most humans did 100 years ago, in the process burning fossil fuels and causing pollution.

Fossil fuel use, air pollution, climate change and health
Every day vast amounts of gasoline, oil, coal and natural gas are combusted. These sources of energy power our industrial society, but burning fossil fuels creates unwanted byproducts. There are

direct health effects; in the UK air pollution is reckoned to aggravate asthma, and lead to an increase of between 12–14,000 deaths from cardio-respiratory disease each year.

Fossil fuel combustion results in the creation of many pollutants, including carbon monoxide, oxides of nitrogen, ozone, sulphur dioxide, volatile organic compounds and small air borne particulates (of particular relevance are those of less than 10 micrometers in diameter—PM10s). Individual pollutants are associated with specific increases in respiratory illness. Although governments may set desirable limits, there are no 'safe' levels for most of the pollutants. As well as contributing to asthma,[28] PM10s have been implicated in lung cancer.[29]

PM10 production has very different profiles in the poor and rich areas of the world. In the rich, PM10 production is associated with a prolific use of energy (particularly from the internal combustion engine and generation of electricity from fossil fuels). In the poor, however, it is associated with energy poverty, as the majority of PM10 production is from burning wood and cow dung. Even a minor reduction in particulates could save millions of lives worldwide.

A 1997 World Bank report concluded that in China alone, if there is no change in fossil fuel consumption rates, related health care costs are likely to leap from $32 billion to $390 billion over the next 20 years. This includes 600,000 premature deaths and 5.5 million cases of chronic bronchitis. A 1996 Ontario (Canada) governmental report calculated that reducing key pollutants by 45% would dramatically reduce hospital admissions and other health costs, resulting in savings of $1 billion annually.

Global warming due to the excessive burning of fossil fuel is also a health risk. It will change agricultural patterns, alter water availability, cause increasing desertification and a substantial rise in sea levels, and extend the habitat of disease-bearing insects. This will cause social, economic and demographic dislocation due to effects on the economy, infrastructure, and supply of resources in many communities. The recent furore in New York over the possible spread into the city of encephalitis carried by mosquitoes is an excellent example of the potential health risks, which in this case were compounded by the addition of many tons of pesticides that were sprayed over the city.

The way of life of those in the rich North is only possible because of the enormous amount of energy we use. It is of course this way of life that predisposes us to most of the diseases that we are now suffering from. The obesogenic, hypermobile consumer society in which heart disease, strokes and many environmentally related cancers flourish, is therefore as closely related to fossil fuel consumption as is climate change. Actions which help reverse climate change will also help slim down the obesogenic society, and so help reduce the prevalence of the diseases of modern consumer societies.

Persistent Organic Pollutants (POPs) and health

Persistent organic pollutants (POPs) and the radioactive materials generated by the nuclear industry are prime pollutants of soil and water, and detrimental to health. POPs are carbon-based chemical compounds and mixtures that include industrial chemicals like PCBs (polychlorinated biphenyls), pesticides like DDT, and unwanted waste byproducts of industry like dioxins. They are so persistent in the environment that they are likely to be present in every living organism on earth.

Even at very low concentrations, POPs have the potential to injure living organisms through the disruption of normal biological functions. They are usually fat-soluble, and so tend to accumulate in the fatty tissues of animals and then concentrate many millions of times as they move up the food chain. The most common route of exposure for humans is through their food. For instance, PCBs and dioxins concentrate in human fat stores causing breast-fed babies to receive particularly high doses.[30] Indeed in Holland women are now being warned against breast feeding their children for more than 6 months, creating a great dilemma since breastmilk is otherwise the ideal food for young babies. Anxiety about this is spreading throughout Europe.

Many POPs have oestrogenic properties, and interfere with hormonal activity. This may explain declining sperm counts and the increasing incidence of hermaphroditism and penile abnormalities. Many POPs are also carcinogenic; dioxins are implicated in bone marrow, lymph gland, lung and muscle cancers, and PCBs are a possible agent in breast cancer. Many have an effect on foetal development, inducing low birth-weight babies. Some are immunosuppressive agents similar to, although not as devastating as, the AIDS virus.

Twelve POPs, nine of which are insecticides, have come under intense scrutiny.[31] The manufacture and use of this 'dirty dozen' has been banned in many countries, and there is international action through the United Nations Environment Program to ban them globally. However, billions of tons of man-made chemicals, most of them inadequately studied despite their known toxicity, have already been manufactured. So the elimination of this dirty dozen is only a start. We must work to ban all POPs.

The case of POPs clearly illustrates the need to adopt the precautionary principle when we are dealing with new developments in science and technology.

Addressing social concerns at the expense of environmental concerns

There is a widespread understanding that social conditions such as poverty undermine health. However, even when these concerns are addressed, it is often at the cost of the environment, with little awareness of the implications that this has. For instance, health workers believe that social reforms in education, housing and welfare benefit (coupled with the provision of clean water and hygienic disposal of sewage) are the main cause of any public health improvements. These gains, largely made in the rich Western societies on the back of wealth created through industrialisation, have usually been made at the cost of our environment. Despite the concerns and promises of the Rio Summit, there remain few governments that are taking serious measures to improve health, without simultaneously damaging the environment.

During the past twenty years, according to the WHO, at least thirty new diseases have emerged to threaten the health of hundreds of millions of people. Environmental changes have contributed to the appearance of most, if not all, of these. The felling of forests and the conversion of grasslands to agricultural lands have directly contributed to such change. In other instances, simple behavioural changes have favoured the emergence of a disease pathogen. For example, new and widespread vector-breeding sites in urban environments have been created through careless disposal of waste.

Conversely, there is no point in improving the local environment if it damages health. In Scandinavia, for example, indoor ventilation has been reduced substantially in many dwellings to save energy, but that has led to increased humidity and prevalence of house dust mites. This in turn has contributed to an increase in childhood asthma and allergies. Similarly, diesel engines were promoted in the UK because of their lower emissions of carbon dioxide compared to conventional petrol engines. However, this led to increased emissions of fine PM10 particles that have been associated with adverse health effects. Environment and health should be seen as two sides of the same coin, and in thinking of one, it is important to review the consequences for the other.

Definitions and markers of environmental sustainability

To prevent environmental degradation and its health consequences, all health-related decisions should be made and developed within the limits of environmental sustainability. At present, we are systematically undermining the sustainability of our environment. In our attempts to reverse the process, we need a clear definition of sustainability and markers to measure our progress.

Sustainability—a working definition

A sustainable physical environment is one that can satisfy today's needs without endangering those of future generations. We all now recognise that sustainability implies that there are limits to the benefits we get from the environment, and thus on the environment's capacity to support our health. There is for instance a limit to the amount of clean water and air available, a limit to the amount of additives or pollutants our air, water and soil can cope with, and a limit to which human intrusion can occur, whilst still preserving space for aesthetics. For the environment to be sustainable we need to live within this limit, to live in balance with nature. The limit for any given substance, or resource, is known as the 'environmental allowance'. If we individually or collectively exceed this allowance, we will erode our physical environment and so ultimately jeopardise our health.

Environmental space and ecological footprints

This environmental allowance is the environmental space each one of us can occupy without causing long term damage. A representation of this is the ecological footprint, which is the area of land required to sustainably provide a person, region or nation with resources (such as food or timber) and absorb their waste (including gases such as CO_2). For instance, each European citizen currently has a footprint of some three hectares, yet worldwide only 1.5

hectares/person of productive land is available. If European figures were applied globally, we would need two planets.[32]

These ideas of environmental space and footprints are relatively new, as is the notion that we are damaging our environment each time we exceed our allowance. At present the effects of the damage are rarely highlighted. We know from previous experience that identifying a new problem is not usually enough. For health workers to take the issue seriously, the problem needs to be named. Therefore the damage that we cause to planetary health by exceeding our environmental space can be called 'Non-accidental Injury to the Planet' (NAIP). We have also given this syndrome an eponym, 'Carson's syndrome', in honour of one of the first scientists to describe our impact on the environment, in her book *Silent Spring*. Carson's syndrome describes the damage done to the environment by the non-sustainable actions of individuals, which is already causing significant health problems. If we don't take Carson's syndrome seriously, and act upon it, the consequences for our individual and collective health will be catastrophic.

Ecological footprints and environmental justice

As sustainability is put at greatest risk by our present energy use, the drive towards the efficient use of energy and towards renewable energy sources is imperative. By reducing our use of fossil fuels, each of us moves towards appropriately sized footprints, and both the local and global environment become cleaner and healthier. Appropriately sized footprints for all the world's inhabitants will constitute environmental justice. For those of us in the rich North the pathway to environmental justice will require us to contract the environmental space that we presently occupy. Thus contraction used in this sense implies a move toward environmental justice.

In summary, a succinct definition of a society in good physical and mental health is therefore one in which the level of social capital is high, the physical environment is health-promoting, and both are developed within environmental footprints that are sustainable. Convergence— the move towards social justice—will have been achieved at the same time as contraction—the move towards environmental justice.

Contraction: how we get there

Contraction is a shorthand for the move to environmental justice. We need to contract our excessive consumption back down to a sustainable footprint. This will improve the environment, and so bene-fit the public's health. But contraction must not take place without convergence (shorthand for the move to social justice) through a more equal sharing of resources.

Pricing mechanisms such as 'polluter pays' and carbon taxes may fall most heavily on those who have little disposable income—the poor. In technical terms, they will be regressive taxes. A regressive tax designed to nurture aspects of health through environment improve-ment may create further poverty, and so undermine other aspects of health. To resolve this problem, some of the money raised through taxation may be used as a direct subsidy to the poor.

An alternative policy is carbon credits. Domestic CO_2 emissions account for around 50% of total carbon dioxide emissions. Each per-son would at the beginning of each year be given the same number of carbon credits. The credits would be in the form of carbon units, each of which would be the equivalent of 1kg of CO_2 emissions. The 50% of CO_2 attributable to public sector and commercial activities would be put on the market to be competed for by the relevant agencies. Initially carbon credits would only be used to buy primary energy sources (petrol, oil, gas and electricity made from non-renewables). As the scheme progressed, every commodity would have a CO_2 amount attached to it. The appropriate amount of each individual's carbon credits would then be used for each transaction. Any extra carbon credits that an individual had left at the end of the year could be traded. This would give a major incentive to activities of all sorts that minimise CO_2 emissions. The total number of carbon credits available would be set by an independent body, and the amounts gradually decreased over a period of 20 years to bring our footprints down to an appropriate size.

As we have spelt out elsewhere in this text, many such changes—such as to local production and consumption cycles, and a move to walking, cycling and using public transport—would have major ben-efits for health through the production of social capital. Thus con-traction would be accompanied by convergence. The two processes would be mutually supportive.

The reorganisation of society necessary for us to bring our foot-prints to appropriate sizes will create social capital, so unfolding a virtuous spiral of change.

Chapter 3

Restoring the Human Scale to Health

"Go to the people / Live amongst them / Start with where they are /
Build on what they have / And when the task is finished /
The mission accomplished / Of the best leaders / The people will say /
We have done it ourselves." Lao Tzu (600 BC)

People change systems

Understanding the social and environmental conditions needed to attain good health is important, but in the end it is changing the system that matters. It is people who generate change. The impetus for involvement comes when people know that *their* values and concerns will underpin and shape the organisation of health. Indeed, the fact these values are largely ignored is an important cause of the problems that lie in our present health systems.

This chapter aims to show that when people's values are incorporated into our health systems, we will be well on the way to gaining health-enhancing social and environmental changes. It is these values that create the vibrant, diverse and sustainable societies from which health springs. But it is only through human scale decision-making and interaction that they can be realised.

The importance of scale to human activities

An understanding of the importance of scale to human activities was at the root of the philosophy of Schumacher and his mentor Leopold Kohr, and it is at the heart of this Briefing. My proposition is that public partnership and engagement will create the type of societies that nourish health. Engagement and partnership flourish when people, and the communities they form through dialogue and interaction, are the focus of decision-making.

A sensible first step to both understanding and promoting dialogue and interaction is to ask the public what it is they want from their health service.[33, 34] Surprisingly, there is not much research on this. The little there is suggests that the public want, and expect, seven basic services ('values') from their health care system. It also suggests that the public understand that these are relevant to both health promotion and health care. If they were in place, both health and health care would be of a high quality.

However, each of these values can only be realised in a health system driven by people who through dialogue and interaction can relate directly to each other. In other words, a human-scale health system. Indeed the move away from this human scale, a feature of most contemporary health care systems, is a major cause of the gulfs identified in Chapter One.

The seven values are as follows:

1. COMPASSIONATE INVOLVEMENT
The public wish to play an active part in the health system they create and the care that they receive. They want information offered with empathy, and care to be given with compassion.

Patients and citizens as agents, not objects
In our present health system, health professionals underestimate the importance of incorporating patients' and citizens' views into consultations—whether relating to health or health care.[35] Health care is often something done to us by professionals rather than being a creative part of our own experience. A renowned patients' advocate puts the situation succinctly, "It's easy to think that patients (and citizens) are for doing things to and for, but they are not—they are for doing things with."[36] As I have said, people should be the agents, not the objects, of health care. Treating patients as objects rather than agents is not a recent problem, but has been developing as medicine has evolved from traditional systems to post-Newtonian 'scientific medicine'.

The different types of knowledge
There is a gap between the perception of health professionals that patients are objects, and citizens who perceive themselves as agents. There is also a parallel gap between the types of knowledge used when health professionals communicate with patients and citizens. In traditional medical systems, the ideas of health and disease were so bound up with the world-view of society that citizens and practi-

tioners shared the same understanding of their health and their illness. *Experiential knowledge* reflecting the lived experience that we all obtain through our direct encounters with illness and health, and *propositional knowledge* based on scientific and theoretical concepts, were closely related. This was also the case for Galenic medicine in Europe. However, as 'scientific medicine' displaced the traditional model, a distance developed between citizens, whose concepts of health and illness were still close to the traditional ideas, and the doctors, who became increasingly mechanistic in their outlook. Over the years, patients began to agree with Voltaire's view that doctors were people who gave medicines about which they knew little, to cure diseases about which they knew less, to people about whom they knew nothing. Whilst this is clearly an overstatement, it reflects people's feelings about the shortcomings of mechanistic medicine. These have fired the increasing interest in traditional medicine that combines the promotion of health with the treatment of disease.

The disconnection and distancing of health providers from the citizenry has caused significant problems for Western scientific medicine, and for our health systems. The problem starts when the patient or citizen tells their story, which is then all too often recast and professionalised, to the detriment of all. The recasting is a consequence of the importance that professionals give to the different types of knowledge. Experiential and *presentational knowledge* (the rich manner in which we recount and explain this experience), are often of less importance to professionals than *propositional knowledge.*[37] Unsurprisingly, propositional knowledge is usually the preserve of the professionals. An effective understanding and treatment of health and disease, however, requires a balanced consideration of information derived from each type of knowledge.

Physicians' own experience
Most physicians recognise the equal importance, and impact, of each type of knowledge to good care when they themselves are ill. For instance, Franz Ingelfinger, an expert on oesophageal cancer, developed the disease himself. He visited a series of experts who gave him information, but not care. It wasn't until he finally visited his family doctor, who knew his circumstances and listened to him as a human being, not a cancer expert, that he got the care he

needed. Similar stories are commonplace among my health colleagues who have suffered a serious illness, and now realise the
dangers of professional dominance. They speak of the importance
to their cure of a shared joke, a touch, and other communication
that reflects the common humanity that binds us. In a recent survey
in the UK,[38] 59% of doctors who had suffered a serious illness said
that it had made them more empathic towards patients.

Communication and empathy

The importance of communication and empathy to the healing and
health-promoting process are acknowledged by all health systems.
Both of these qualities are heavily dependent on the relationship
between patient and healer, regardless of whether the interaction is
to cure disease or promote health. Some of us conventional doctors
have marginalised these concerns, and this is the cause of many of
the complaints directed at us by our patients. "Conventional health
professionals don't pay enough attention to good communication"
is a frequent criticism also levelled at us by complementary therapists
(see Box 8). Fortunately, universities are encouraging an emphasis on
patient-doctor communication in the medical syllabus, and also
introducing courses on complementary therapies. Both of these
approaches may help, but we still have a long way to go. For
although individual health workers usually display the essential qualities of dignity, compassion and equity in their work, modern health
systems (whether curative or preventive) are dominated by health
professionals and are not imbued with the human interactions
needed to make them work.

Supportive communication and patient involvement

To move towards a more human-scale and compassionate interaction
between professionals and patients, the technological expertise of the
professionals should be integrated with patients' and citizens' views.
This task requires clear and supportive communication during the consultation. I am always gratified by the relief of my patients when I make
it explicit that whatever the outcome of our consultation, I will be honest to them about the findings. Such communication does not always
occur. For example, there is a widespread perception that health care
professionals undertake more investigations and initiate more treatments than the patients themselves would wish.

Box 8: The growth of complementary and alternative medicine

What is complementary medicine?
Complementary and alternative medicine (CAM) is a process that 'complements' the patient at physical, mental, emotional and spiritual levels. The term CAM covers a very broad range of treatments including Chinese medicine, reflexology, osteopathy, acupuncture, chiropractice, yoga and psychotherapy. In the 1970s and 1980s these disciplines were seen as an alternative to conventional health care, and became known as 'alternative medicine'. Lately, as the two systems have begun to be used alongside (to 'complement') each other, the term complementary medicine is used. The aim of CAM is to bring the vital force and spirit back into line with the balance of the body to allow a return to wholeness.

Conventional doctors are deemed to use a reductionist approach in their healing. By contrast, CAM practitioners are credited with taking a more holistic view, and examining the whole range of emotional, spiritual and environmental factors that influence a patient's condition. However, there are many well-loved conventionally trained practitioners, whose practice is as rounded as complementary therapists. Many of these welcome the increasing popular interest in complementary medicine, anticipating that public pressure will reorientate all healing toward the best practice in both systems.

On the increase
Increasing availability of, and demand for, CAM is evidence of its popularity. A recent study in Australia showed that a fifth of the population had seen a complementary practitioner in the previous year, and nearly half had used some form of complementary treatment. In France, where homeopathy is most popular form of CAM, its use rose from 16% of the population in 1982 to 36% in 1992.[39] This suggests that in some countries CAM is now an established pattern of care alongside other models of health.

The number and profile of complementary practitioners is changing rapidly. In 1981 about 13,500 registered practitioners were working in the UK. In only sixteen years this figure had trebled to about 40,000, with three disciplines—healing, aromatherapy and reflexology—accounting for over half of all registered complementary practitioners. Meanwhile interest from conventionally trained doctors is also rising. Recent figures for the UK showed that over a third of general practitioners had received training in complementary therapies, with 15-42% wanting further training.

Box 8 (continued)

Attention to personality and personal experience

Patient surveys show that the most intense reaction is usually an exasperation at the failure of conventional medicine to satisfactorily address their condition. CAM can offer hope to such patients, both by attempting to influence the underlying disease and, often more importantly, by addressing emotional states, energy levels, coping styles, and other aspects that contribute to quality of life. This is particularly important for patients with chronic diseases and no prospect of cure from conventional medicine (e.g. cancer, HIV infection and multiple sclerosis). Surveys show that this group of people use CAM up to twice as much as the general population.

Other reasons cited for the increase in use of CAM are the growing perception of the limitations of orthodox treatments and increasing concerns about its side effects, reliance on technology, and invasive techniques.[40] The brevity of conventional medicine consultations, lack of rapport with the doctor, and a feeling of having a treatment imposed without adequate explanation, has also been mentioned.

Patients seem to appreciate the time and attention they receive during a CAM consultation, the ways in which their illness is explained, and the environment in which they receive treatment. CAM also encourages patients to explain their experience and understanding of their problem, which in itself can be therapeutic. Some CAM users cite the increased opportunities for active participation in the process of recovery as a reason for choosing complementary medicine. There is also a greater use of physical contact in CAM than in conventional medicine, which brings a less distancing and more human experience to health care. It can also build an open and honest rapport between practitioners and patients, and help the healing process.

Some patients have existential concerns that conventionally trained professionals may not feel competent to address. These range from the otherwise healthy adolescent who can find no meaning in life to the terminally ill patient confronting his or her own mortality. Many complementary disciplines make no distinction between spiritual and other symptoms, and offer treatments aimed at all aspects of a person's life or illness.

Consumer surveys consistently show how positive public attitudes are to CAM, with about 60% of the public in the Netherlands and Belgium declaring themselves ready to pay extra health insurance premiums for it, and 74% of the British public favouring it being available on the NHS.[41]

Patient involvement in decision-making
It needs to be acknowledged that patient views and priorities must be taken more seriously. Patients do want more time in consultations: this will have resource implications for a patient-sensitive health service. But when this time allows for sharing of information and explanations which are accessible to the patients, services are used more appropriately (and often less).

- Patients with prostate problems often choose the watch and wait option, not surgery.[42]
- Patients who have acute lower respiratory tract illness can manage their own illness if they are given the requisite information.[43]
- Patients with physical symptoms that remain unexplained after one year benefit enormously from explanations which resonate with their own understanding of the cause of their illness. These empowering explanations help recovery and reduce their use of the health service.[44]
- Patients with breast cancer do not always wish for chemotherapy, even when health workers think it might prolong their lives.
- Advanced Directives. People who make these directives usually do so to ensure that they are not given life-prolonging care when the quality of their lives will be unacceptable to them (see Box 9).

The citizen's voice: Advanced Directives
One way of ensuring that patients' views are heard is through the use of Advanced Directives (ADs), sometimes called 'Living Wills'. These statements afford people the opportunity to predetermine treatment were they to suffer from defined categories of illness. For example, if a patient had a severe stroke, or became mentally and physically incompetent, they could have used an AD to have expressed their treatment preferences prior to the illness (see Box 9). I myself have written an AD. The control of the direction of treatment by the patient through ADs, or by any other means, would reduce the amount of suffering and also resource use.

There is increasing interest in these documents, but little formal research into their impact. More research on their acceptability would help to clarify the implications. However, if patients are to make considered judgements about the amount of care they want, there has to be public confidence that such decisions by health care professionals, whilst taking cost into account, are not solely made on a financial basis. So a trusting relationship between health professionals and citizens is a necessary first step in the delivery of empathic care.

2. COLLECTIVE DECISION-MAKING
The public wish to influence the range of health and health care that they receive from the General Practice or hospital.

The democratic deficit in health
The situation at present in many health systems is that decision-makers are increasingly distanced from the impact of their decisions—both geographically and socially—and don't experience their results. 'Moral blunting' (our capacity to insulate ourselves from the consequences of decisions which we make but are not subject to), is an inevitable consequence. When making rationing and other difficult decisions, moral blunting makes it easier to adopt an attitude of, "let them eat cake." We have forgotten an important guideline for moral action: "do as you would be done by".

For instance, in the UK's present health service neither the local health authorities (the purchasers of care), nor the various NHS Trusts and General Practitioners (the providers of care), engage effectively with their constituencies—despite the fact that there are local representatives on boards, and consultation is widespread. These efforts are often no more than token gestures, and many commentators have spoken about the democratic deficit in health.[46]

Human scale health—the importance of local decision-making
One way of bringing the human scale into focus in decision-making is to bring the process to a more local level. Local decisions that impact equally on the local decision-makers and the community are likely to be more morally acute. The present situation is characterised by central authorities determining which decisions can be permitted locally. Enlightened authorities may pass more, rather than less, decisions to the local community, but ultimately the right to decide remains with the centre, rather than with the periphery. This process should be reversed, in order to infuse humanity back into health care, to move away from the present fragmentation of services and towards reciprocity and co-operation (see Box 10).

Box 9: Advanced Directives (ADs)

Advanced Directives (or 'Living Wills') are statements made in advance of an illness about the type and extent of treatment a person would want, on the assumption that they may be incapable of participating in decision-making about treatment at the time. For many people the ultimate horror is not death, but to be maintained in limbo in a hospital or nursing home by machines controlled by strangers. This scenario is all too common in the health services of the rich democracies. I (like many of my colleagues) have informally asked patients and friends what their view of such an eventuality is. The overwhelming response is that if they became incapable of meaningful communication, they would wish only to have comfort care—no life-prolonging interventions.

Thus there is a dilemma, as the approach that is often promoted by both relatives and doctors is one of intervention. This is pursued on the grounds that staying alive is the only goal. In other circumstances they would not be able to override the wishes of the patient.

Luis Kutner, a Chicago attorney, drew up the first AD in 1967. This document gave instructions about medical care in the last few days of life. The central tenet was that the signatories did not want their life prolonged once they became unable to express their own wishes directly. ADs aim to put the patients' wishes centre stage again.

Inevitably in such a sensitive area, the legal status of these directives has developed unevenly. Denmark provides us with a good model, as ADs have been made legally binding, and there is a central computer-based registry of those who have written them. In 1996, the UK decided not to enact legislation. This failure to legislate reflected the views of a House of Lords committee: that patients are best served by relying on the recognised duty of physicians to provide only that treatment to an incompetent patient that is both reasonable and in the interests of that patient.

Local communities determine where decisions are made
The starting point is that individuals working in and together with their local communities should have the right to make all decisions relating to their health and health care. These groups may well decide that some health functions will need to straddle a number of communities. Decisions about these functions can then be passed to a community of the appropriate size to implement them. Thus the local group of people will pass on decisions to other levels, where they feel it to be nec-

essary. The essence of this framework is that local people determine the appropriate level for decision-making, and so the scale at which differing health decisions take place is passed up from below, not down from above. The scale of decision-making is determined by groups of people who are able to communicate directly with one another, and who will be the direct beneficiaries of the decisions made. Thus the scale, whilst not exclusively local, is always determined by the local people.

Techniques for engaging the public
To realise our goal of a health system built on the experiential knowledge of citizens, the many techniques now available for engaging with the public need to be utilised. For instance, in Lewisham, London, I have been involved with our local council in running a citizen's panel. This randomly selected group of citizens has demonstrated to me that asking local people for their input into local services has real value. However, the citizens' voice, in the form of patient user groups or pressure groups, usually raises concerns about improving services and introducing new ones.

Consequences of community-based decision-making
An important consequence of this local, human-scale, community-based decision-making in health and health care is the plurality and diversity of provision that would inevitably arise. Different communities will have different priorities, and will seek to make change at different rates. This reflects the assets that each individual community has and so is, in principle, to be welcomed; but what if one community makes decisions that are at odds with the prevailing socially accepted norms, or if a community in the UK decided for instance, to curtail women's access to abortion? One of the arguments for uniformity of provision of health is to minimise variations in care across the country, and to guard against perverse variations at a local level. One simple solution is the enactment of a bill of rights and responsibilities to both other humans and the environment. This would act as a safeguard against excess, and so ensure that diversity and plurality enhanced the human and environmental condition. However, localities might explore other ways of ensuring that 'local' doesn't come to mean 'blinkered'. Mediators from other localities could be used to help resolve disputes about priorities, and links and exchanges between localities could be arranged. Both these actions would constitute a form of peer review.

Box 10: Urban governance and health development in León, Nicaragua[46]

Nicaragua is an extremely poor country, and is characterised by social, political and epidemiological polarisation. León is the country's second largest city, with nearly 200,000 inhabitants, 60% of whom live in conditions of poverty and 24% in conditions of extreme deprivation. Unemployment levels are close to 60%, and in the past two decades, rapid urban growth has led to a rise in slums. In many areas the basic prerequisites for health, such as safe water, sanitation, electricity and waste disposal, are lacking.

León has a history of citizen participation, a strong community-based organisation—the Movimiento Comunal—and an effective model of local governance. Following the 1986 elections, a number of organisations proposed strengthening citizen participation in policy-making, developing an integrated approach to public health problems, and improving living conditions and the environment. This was the start of the León healthy municipalities' initiative—part of the World Health Organisation's Healthy Cities project.

The local development commission launched policies to ensure the basic prerequisites for health in the city. Strategies have been introduced to reduce the illiteracy rate, provide safe and adequate water supplies, build and improve housing, control waste water and ensure the adequate disposal of waste. With the co-operation of the local media and the city's primary schools, problems of violence and issues related to mental health have also been addressed.

From the beginning, this initiative has gone beyond purely providing health services. It has placed health at the centre of sustainable local and national development, which in turn has created many effective alliances between the community, local government, local organisations, the university and other stakeholders. This has led to increased opportunities for local citizens to participate in decision-making, and ultimately has given them real power over the decisions that affect their lives, and their health.

In November 1998 a tragedy struck Nicaragua—hurricane Mitch—and tested the capacity of León's community to respond. In the first few days, brigades of hundreds of volunteers were mobilised and sent to the most affected areas, while the limited resources at the local level were made available to the local authorities. It has been argued that the model of urban governance and the healthy municipality initiative were instrumental in providing an immediate response and in addressing the basic needs of the population in the wake of the disaster.

3. BEST PRACTICE
The public wishes care to be based on the best scientific and technological evidence available.

Clinical decision-making
There are large areas of medical practice in which clinical decision-making is not, and perhaps cannot be, based on data which has established the effectiveness of the intervention. These grey zones of clinical practice range from hysterectomies, which are judged to be of uncertain value in 25% of cases, to coronary angioplasty, where the figure is 38%.[47] Even where there is established evidence, based on randomised control trials (in perhaps 30% of medical interventions), this doesn't always guide the actions of clinicians. Part of the problem of implementing so-called 'best-practice' is that citizens' contributions have seldom been incorporated into the evaluation of treatments; thus evaluation is not based on an appropriate balance and range of knowledge and experience.[48] Treatment based on more balanced evidence would be likely to result in a reduction in the present rate of interventions. This could release sufficient resources to cover the cost of introducing new services, as well as to fund some of the presently unmet demand.

Clinical research
Patients and citizens are valuable sources of information and collaboration for research. Patients who have suffered a particular disease, or who have undergone certain treatments, have experience and skills that complement those of clinical researchers. At present, it is rare that they are consulted as to which research questions are worth asking, and when a question should be framed differently. One example of a successful research project that did involve patient input, and changed management procedures, was carried out at the Mount Vernon Hospital in the USA. Researchers had hypothesised that moving follow-up breast cancer clinics to primary care might relieve the burden on hospital outpatient clinics. However, the project was redesigned to address the issue of easier access to specialists, after researchers consulted with women who had experienced problems with the new arrangements.[49]

In Chapter Two, the interventions needed to improve health were discussed. The evidence base for their efficacy is rather better than that for much of the health care we practice. Little effort, however, is made to implement this knowledge. Not many health professionals will for instance seriously consider the impact their institutions have on narrowing the gap between the rich and the poor of their communities. If a health facility used its purchasing power to ameliorate relative poverty, it could have an enormous impact on health.

4. MANAGERIAL COMPETENCE
The public value care that is well organised.

The role of citizens' groups
To ensure organisational efficiency, experiential knowledge must be used as the basis for change. There are an increasing number of individuals and user organisations providing such knowledge to the health service and to the community groups active in health promotion. For instance, the citizens' panel in Lewisham, London, helped redesign the patient information booklet to make it much more user-friendly and accessible, and patient pressure helped us to relocate all cancer services into one geographical site, with immediate practical benefits to patients. These are welcome advances, but the organisation of much health care is still based on propositional knowledge, often gained through time and management surveys.

A shift of resources
Appropriate organisation could substantially reduce the resources that are used to deliver the present level of care. For example, patients in a hospital very often have to repeat the same information about themselves to different departments. Does this make a patient feel central to the process, or merely an adjunct to bureaucracy? Is this the most efficient use of resources? To improve the infrastructure and information technology capacity, capital investment would be necessary.

In the UK, for example, over the last twenty years there has been a substantial shift of health care from hospitals to the community and General Practice (where 92% of contacts now take place), but there hasn't been an equivalent devolution in decision-making and finances. This must now happen. Only then can an engaged citizenry, informed by trusted health workers, use its resources to organise health care to its own specifications. This reorganisation will ensure that care presently delivered in district hospitals will be available at local community hospitals, with highly specialised care being concentrated in fewer specialist hospitals.

5. APPROPRIATE TRAINING
The public value health professionals who are well trained, and whose research is relevant to our problems.

Involving citizens
Patients often complain that health workers don't give patient-friendly information, and that they don't undertake relevant research. Citizens are now involved in ethics committees that approve research, and are represented on major committees that grant research money, but there is still a lack of public involvement in determining the range and direction of research topics, and the content of the under- and post-graduate curriculum. My experience in Zimbabwe of negotiating with local people over a research project which they wanted undertaken, and which we were able to perform, showed me how valuable this way of controlling and conducting research can be. The local people outside Harare had a high prevalence of goitre (enlarged thyroid). Although this was not their first health priority, when they heard that we had the necessary expertise to investigate the causes of this illness they helped design and run the project. Patients going to traditional healers also welcomed the research that we carried out with these healers.

Although many clinicians value involving patients in medical education, and my teaching sessions involving patients are always more instructive, there has been little formal recognition of this in syllabus design. So the educational opportunities for promoting communication and mutual understanding between professionals and patients has been insufficiently developed. As well as this lack of citizen input, there has been a woeful lack of investment in training for many of the staff working in a health care environment. There is no doubt that to achieve an improvement in training, including incorporating the views and skills of citizens and patients, would cost extra money.

Box 11: Environmental and Social Impact Assessment (ESIA)

A growing number of commercial, public and voluntary organisations are assessing their social and environmental impacts (for example The Body Shop, Shell and British Telecom). Their yearly financial auditing is complemented by a report on the social and environmental issues raised by their activities. These issues must reflect the concerns of all the stakeholders. In industry, the pressing reason for these audits is the recognition that productivity is increased when staff feel valued and involved in decisions about all aspects of their work. The health service has an additional motive—in demonstrating that ESIAs are good for health as well as productivity.

As all aspects of our physical and social environment play important parts in determining our health, the need to investigate and monitor them is self-evident. Indeed, when societies put health rather than wealth at the centre of their aspirations, ESIA and Health Impact Assessment (HIA) will be the same. The aim of HIAs, and increasingly of ESIAs, is to be able to estimate the impact of a specified policy on the health of the defined population.

Take hospitals, for example: because of the numbers of people employed, the health and welfare of staff make a significant contribution to health statistics. Furthermore, hospitals should be healthy organisations, which necessarily implies a concern with their social and environmental performance. Hospitals, and indeed all other health care institutions, should be advocates for health, not only for those that work in and use them, but more widely too.

Hospitals do not at present have a mechanism for assessing whether they fulfil this role, and I believe that ESIA is presently the best available mechanism. Examples of issues which should be covered in such an assessment are:

- The degree to which staff feel fully engaged with the setting of goals and running of the organisation.
- The extent to which staff feel they work in an organisation which enjoys 'power with', not 'power over' leadership.
- The physical environment (for instance noise, warmth and comfort).
- Issues of energy usage and waste disposal.
- The way in which the institution supports its immediate environment, through employment and purchasing power, and use of the facilities by the local citizens.
- The extent to which all the above ensure that patients get a better quality of care.

6. A HEALTHY HEALTH CARE ENVIRONMENT
The public wish that the health care environment is itself health-promoting.

Health institutions should have workplace policies and physical environments that are therapeutic, with a sustainable energy and waste policy. This would offer staff a working environment that was 'health sustaining' rather than 'health draining'. Institutions that delivered health care in this exemplary fashion would, of course, be health promoting, and so would bridge the gap between delivering health care and actually improving the health of the local population.

Environmental and social impact assessments (ESIAs) as tools for health
Although there has been an emphasis on health at work, this tends to concentrate on the prevention of accidents and anti-smoking and anti-drinking campaigns. The participative techniques of ESIAs, which are designed to seek people's views on their workplace, share best practice from across all workplaces, and start redesigning based on these views, have not as yet been used in hospitals or general practice. However, together with colleagues, I am involved in such a project in Lewisham hospital.

The proper introduction of ESIAs is a good first step in defining how to achieve a healthy workplace, and could lead to major savings (see Box 11). For instance, the consequences of an ESIA might be to radically reduce staff sickness (presently around 6% in the UK) to the level of best practice (around 2%) and energy costs by 50%— neither of them impossible tasks. These measures could save at least a billion pounds each year from the National Health Service budget. As the workforce would also be healthier, the cost of any treatment that they might incur would also be saved, as well as the money spent on employing temporary staff to cover sick leave. Money would also be saved on apparently simple problems like water wastage, which costs the NHS £40,000,000 per year.

ESIAs can be used at an individual, household, community, national and even international level. At each level the assessment will help us define what the prevailing level of health is, and what we need to do to improve things. To make the necessary changes that such an assessment will identify will however need capital investment (for example in energy conservation, renewable energy development, and the improvement of working and living conditions), and all of this requires social and political will, as well as long term vision.

7. FINANCIAL PRUDENCE
The public wish to ensure that their care is delivered in as cost effectively as possible.

Future financial pressures
The introduction of each of the above mentioned values would lead to effective use of money. However there are undoubtedly additional pressures on health care systems that an engaged citizenry will have to confront. Indeed, all rich democracies are facing mounting pressure on their health care budgets. Conventional wisdom has it that this pressure will get worse, as:

- the number of dependent people is going to increase (the demography of an ageing population) and they are going to need increasing health care;
- with an ageing population, it is likely that there will be a decreasing number of people in full or part time work paying taxes;
- the nature of technological advance increases the range and sophistication of treatments available to us all; and
- there will be an increasing mismatch between expectation and resources.

Some of the above pressures may be ameliorated by measures being put in place to sustain health (for instance by the elimination of poverty), but at the moment, the emphasis is still on treating ill health: 'cure not prevention'. Some of the other pressures may turn out to be overemphasised. For instance, if elderly people are looked after in their local community using local resources, and a LETS or Time Money economy is used, the increased burden of care imposed by the elderly would be very much reduced (see Box 3). Other pressures could be mitigated by an engaged citizenry being involved in decisions about health care. Nevertheless more money, particularly for capital investment, may well be needed. This should not constitute a significant problem, for numerous public surveys suggest that the public wish to invest more money in health care, and in other health-promoting areas such as education and the relief of poverty. This public commitment is not reflected in public expenditure—a good example of the inadequacy of consultation and of the lack of sensitivity of the democratic process.

There should still be a reserve mechanism in place if costs do increase. For instance, the allocation of governmental revenue between the various departments should be explored. If, in the pursuit of our open, engaged society, local people were consulted, money in the defence budget might be reduced and the surplus redirected into health. The possibility of individuals paying for parts of their health care, or raising local taxes to pay for additional local services, could also be addressed through the imaginative use of local money.

Motivating and empowering people

People want to know that once they have articulated their values, they will be listened to, and able to change their circumstances. What, therefore, must we do to give people the capacity to transform their experience of health?

Increasingly the range, remoteness and complexity of the social and physical factors that can cause ill health mean that both health professionals and patients feel unable to control, or change, the situation. For instance, many of my patients recognise that their asthma may be related to pollutants, their acute diarrhoea a result of defects in our agricultural system or food processing, and their depression due to redundancy. However, they can feel powerless to do anything about the causes of their ill health.

Public engagement

We have argued strongly that public engagement in the health care process is a precondition for change. Here the scale of activities is particularly important. Engaging the public demands dialogue and interaction, based on responsible, balanced partnerships. Shared decision-making and budgetary control are essential elements of true partnership, and thus only possible through human scale interactions, most of which must necessarily occur at a local level. Each transaction should be sealed by appropriate contractual obligations and facilitated by supportive management (discussed later). Further, to ensure that local people continue to have input into decisions that relate to larger communities, locals must determine which decisions are passed to a larger community. When decisions affecting people's lives are devolved, the implications are likely to be as relevant to those who

Box 12: Agenda 21 in action—
The MAMA-86 drinking water quality project in the Ukraine

The Agenda 21 document was agreed at the 1992 Earth Summit in Rio, and has been endorsed by over 175 governments. It examines the inter-connectedness of societal, economic and environmental issues and calls for action at local, regional and national levels to make the transition towards sustainability.

The MAMA-86 project was initiated in 1997 after consultations with women community leaders in the Ukraine. Participants considered health, environment and economics the most pressing issues for Ukrainian women, and drinking water was identified as a key issue for action.

Drinking water supply in the Ukraine is affected by intensive pollution of surface and ground water. Many health problems are considered to be associated with the poor water quality, and in some regions water short-age is a problem. Prevalent health problems in towns with highly con-taminated tap water include respiratory, skin and gastro-intestinal diseases, allergies, depression and blood disorders.

In the Ukraine, as in most of the post-Soviet countries, there is no tra-dition of disclosing information or co-operating with the non-govern-mental sectors or consumers. It is difficult for the public to get clear information from official sources about water quality. Above all, there is a need for the public to know how to protect themselves and their families from the health risks associated with inadequate water. In 1997, in the face of this confusion and lack of information, MAMA-86—a community-based women's NGO—undertook their own independent tests on tap water. In addition, due to lack of data MAMA-86 initiated research into public attitudes and habits regarding drinking water. The two research documents represent the first attempt by local independent organisations to collect their own data on water quality. The data successfully drew public attention to the issues, and has set the scene for a more open and informed debate between the different sectors, government and public.

MAMA-86 subsequently invited representatives from water authorities to a seminar to hear the results of their independent research. Many offi-cials attended who had never previously co-operated with NGOs, and most of them made their own data available for inspection. For the first time many citizens had access to the authorities, and opportunities to communicate and share their knowledge. The networking was highly con-structive and has already proved fruitful. MAMA-86 has made the first steps towards achieving cleaner water, by facilitating an integrated

Box 12 (continued)

approach to discussions on drinking water—the key to health for many people in the Ukraine.

This project demonstrates the use of the Agenda 21 initiative to mobilise locally for joint action on health and the environment.

make the decisions as to those who benefit from them. The resultant human-scale interactions will help ensure that any change is owned by the community, and is therefore likely to be both easier to carry through and more enduring.

The issue for a health system that reflects these values and is an integral part of a society in which social and environmental justice prevails is not whether but how the public can most effectively become engaged. There are two distinct aspects of this public engagement:

1. The need for citizens to work directly with one another, working as agents of change, to create the social and physical community which we have outlined in Chapter Two (see Box 12).

2. The role of citizens acting as advocates in order to remove the structural impediments to social and environmental improvements. Given that there are impediments in a number of social and environmental areas, citizen advocacy will need to cover a wide range of topics, as demonstrated by Jubilee 2000 (see Box 13).

Given the array of problems blocking our path to good health, citizen advocacy will need to be pervasive and persuasive. Considerable public pressure will have to be deployed to force the changes necessary to reverse social injustice and create social capital whilst not exceeding our environmental limit. For instance, enabling more people to be usefully employed, to have greater degree of control over their lives, to use public transport, to walk and cycle, and reduce the need to travel will all require many structural changes in the organisation of our societies. Perhaps the most important of these changes is the creation of opportunities for local decision-making so that citizens can control their own destinies. Many of these structural changes will require action at many levels, and all changes should ideally improve both the social and environmental situation. There are plenty of good examples of the potential of such change, three of which are now explored:

Box 13: Jubilee 2000

Health workers need to be involved in a wider understanding of the determinants of good health in order to change these for the better. Many of these determinants have been identified in the text. Poverty, leading to a limited access to resources, is one of the determinants that is profoundly detrimental to health. The international debt of the third world, which exacerbates poverty among the already poor, is a clear example of an apparently economic problem that has major social, environmental and health effects. In essence, the debt is due to the inability of many poor countries to repay either interest on capital or loans made to their governments in the 1970s. The debt repayment is at the cost of the poorest people in poor countries. Whoever is responsible for the making and taking of loans in the first instance, it's certainly not them.

Medact, the UK organisation for health workers who wish to promote health through eradicating social and economic injustices, has been campaigning for debt relief since 1987. It was a founder member of the Campaign Against the Debt Network that was renamed Jubilee 2000 in 1995.

The coalition Jubilee 2000 is composed of the Churches and many NGOs, in addition to Medact. Medact's specific role is to give the health perspective; to articulate why it is that the debt is so damaging to the social cohesion and environmental sustainability that are essential to good health. The coalition has been enormously influential in raising international concern about the debt. One of the most powerful influences has been explaining to the public the impact of debt on health. Thus health workers, many working through Medact, have exerted effective leverage at a national and international level. Colleagues in the World Bank have said that Jubilee 2000 has had a powerful impact on bank thinking. Moreover, the campaign has grabbed the public's attention and has been supported by many citizens' groups across the world, as well as across issues and movements. As a result, many governments have pledged to cancel all or part of their debts with the third world.

1. Creating sustainable footprints
Most of the Western world's footprints are at an unsustainable level—way beyond our environmental limits. However, many of the measures necessary to return them to a sustainable level will both improve the physical environment and create social capital. Examples of this synergy are the creation of work within a local community which would come from programmes to conserve energy and from the generation and use of renewable energy—key requirements if we are to reduce air pollution and CO_2 production.

2. Reversing the dehumanising scale of globalisation
Globalisation of the economy has profound effects on local communities, with associated health consequences. The problems again relate to scale, this time the dehumanising scale of global activities. Whilst global economic activity may well increase the overall amount of wealth generated, there is seldom congruity between the community in which the wealth is generated and that in which its benefits are felt. The environmental damage attributable to globalisation also falls unevenly on different communities. Local communities need to be enabled to use locally generated wealth locally. Time money, LETS schemes, and legislation to prevent asset removal must be in place, and local control is necessary to ensure that it is. Local cycles are much more likely to be environmentally friendly, and where they are not, the damage is more easily identified and rectified.

3. Reorienting global spending patterns
The global pattern of spending also has major impacts for a local community. For instance the annual global subsidy for unsustainable agriculture, fossil fuels, nuclear energy, roads, water and fishing is estimated to be $2,000 billion, and the annual expenditure on armaments is roughly $700 billion. Yet it would cost only $20 billion annually to provide education, basic health care, family planning, food and safe water to all the peoples of the world. It is difficult to believe that local decision-makers would allow such inappropriate profligacy. An important task for local decision-makers is to link local action, often involving personal change, to global action.

Each of the above examples can only be achieved through local people taking control of their destiny. Making this happen will not be easy. Vigorous advocacy will be needed to alter the present centrist and professionally-dominated mind set, which is pervasive not only in our health services but more widely in society. This advocacy will have to be sustained, for as well as changing minds we will need to change the way we organise our societies, a matter we return to in Chapter Four.

Health benefits of the process of engagement

This type and degree of engagement, essential for our purpose, has itself a predictable health benefit. It is likely to create social capital through the formation of networks of people. The process itself is health-promoting. Further, a strong motivational force in the behaviour of adults is to ensure that their children are well catered for. Respected local health professionals are in a strong position to persuade adults of the importance to their children of creating the social and environmental conditions for good health.

Changes in management style

I have shown how the appropriate provision of each of the values citizens wish for from their health system requires the active participation of a committed citizenry. This cannot occur unless there is an appropriate management style and leadership. At present, there is often a divide between 'command and control' (power over, decision-imposing) leadership, and 'creative' (power with, decision-supporting) leadership in the health service, and indeed in the institutions concerned with health outside the conventional health system. For instance, over the last twenty years in the UK there have been some innovative reforms within the health service, yet the opportunities that these offered have often been squandered because the framework for decision-making has not changed: ministers still have to 'defend each fall of a bedpan'.[50] Most of our present health services still have 'power over' management whilst trying to deliver a 'power with' agenda, which is a significant divide; and although health managers are beginning to talk a great deal about partnership working, for this to happen those working together should have equal power. Other services important to health have the same managerial styles.

Examining the evolution of projects within any service gives an indication of management style. Projects in which leaders take 'power with' people have different characteristics to those in which leaders take 'power over' people. The table below gives a useful summary of the differences between the two types of project. If the aim is to

Box 14: The Lewisham MacMillan team—a model of co-operative development

The National Society for Cancer Relief (NSCR), founded in 1911, started by giving financial support to cancer sufferers. However, over the years it became clear that too many people were dying with intolerable burdens of psychological, spiritual and physical pain, and that not only money but more effective palliative care was needed. The hospice movement, energised in the 1960s, began to show that support from trained health professionals could readily provide such care. However many cancer sufferers wished to die at home, and the NSCR began to train specialist 'MacMillan' nurses, who by working between hospitals and the community, were able to support patients at home.

In 1982, the first MacMillan nurses were recruited to Lewisham, London. Their remit was to support individual cancer patients through their journey, ensuring that their personal needs were recognised and addressed. However, there was considerable resistance to these new professionals. Many traditionally trained health professionals felt that specialist nurses should not 'take over' their role in cancer treatment. Moreover doctors took poorly to being advised by nurses.

Undaunted, the MacMillan nurses, working as a collective without hierarchy, identified a few champions in the hospital, and set about showing how they could make a difference. The team approach was to talk with, and respect the views of, other health professionals involved in an individual patient's care. They also acted in a non-adversarial way as patient advocates, introduced new protocols for pain relief, and networked with all the relevant agencies who might be involved in care—but at no stage imposed their views. By demonstrating their ability to improve cancer care, they built a firm base of respect among patients, local general practitioners, and increasingly among the hospital-based consultants. The MacMillan team is now universally recognised as playing a vital role not only in cancer care but also in educating doctors and medical and nursing students in the necessary skills.

engage people in a creative way, there is little room for type B projects. The local MacMillan cancer support team with which I work was developed along type A lines, and has transformed the care of patients dying of cancer within our district (see Box 14). The community development approach to health is predicated on type A management. Only when the health system is infused with leadership and projects characterised by a 'power with' approach, will the health and health care be underpinned by the values and qualities to which we aspire.

Characteristics of projects with different power sharing [51]

PROJECT CHARACTERISTICS	POWER WITH (A)	POWER OVER (B)
Initiated:	Locally	Centrally
Began with:	Action	Plan
Design:	Evolving, Collaborative	Static, Expert
Use of technology:	Indigenous/Scientific	Scientific
Primary Resource Base:	Local people and their assets	Central funds and technicians
Treatment of error:	Embraced	Buried
Supporting organisations:	Built from within the community	Existing, or built from outside
Growth:	Gradual, organic, flexible	Rapid, mechanistic, target-orientated
Staff development:	Continuous, action based	Intermittent, and formal classroom
Organised by:	Teams	Technical experts
Evaluation:	Self-evaluation, continuous	External, intermittent
Leadership:	Strong, sustained, individual	Limited, changing, positional
Duration:	Unlimited	Time limited

Chapter 4

The Reorientation of Health Care Systems

There is no tomorrow—we have to invent it."
Gustav Berger, French philosopher

How far is it possible to change a health care system so that the development of a healthy society becomes as ingrained into the system as the delivery of health care? Using the insights and wisdom of traditional health systems, and building on the requirements for both health and health care that have been described in this briefing, we need to construct a better system for sustaining health in the 21st century:

- where health is viewed holistically, and rooted in a just physical and social environment
- where individual physiological, psychological and spiritual fulfillment flourishes
- where appropriate scale is decided by the people themselves, not a remote bureaucracy
- where leaders exercise 'power with' rather than 'over' people
- where communities are on top, professionals on tap
- where the central value of local agencies and groups is the health prosperity, not the economic prosperity, of the community
- where communities pursue health and hope for wealth, rather than pursuing wealth in the illusion that health will follow.

Current developments

The possibility that we can create such societies is, I believe, better than ever before. People across the world are increasingly well informed about health. Governments have to respond to this new awareness, and changes in thinking are evident at every level. For instance:

- the WHO now recognises that good health is a prerequisite for economic stability, and that improving economic wealth does not necessarily mean better health;

- the European Union has amalgamated several directorates to get a concerted action around the environment, social factors and health;
- the European Environmental Health Action Plan 1994 calls upon every nation to develop a National Environmental Health Action Plan (NEHAP) that is linked to the WHO's Charter on Environment and Health;
- the first international conference on environment and health, where the interactions between social and environmental factors and health were explored, was held in London in June 1999; and
- Local Agenda 21 activities all over the world link health to social and environmental improvements.

Core values and principles

The popular understanding of what constitutes health is universal, as are the core values and principles that should underpin the way in which organisations dedicated to improving health develop their direction and their governance. All reflect the requirements for health that have been outlined. These core values and principles are summarised below.

1. Promotion of health should be at the centre of policy-making. Each initiative undertaken should show how it promotes the health and wellbeing of individuals and/or the population.

2. The new organisations should have the capacity to influence decisions on the many environmental and social issues that underpin health.

3. Although the system will not have wealth promotion as its central aim, a substantial proportion of the rewards of local economic activity should remain in the locality.

4. All decisions should be made locally. Local people may decide to co-operate or collaborate with other partners, but the decision to initiate such collaboration should remain with the local decision-making body. Although there are different scales at which different aspects of health need to be addressed, health-related decisions should regain and retain a human face. For this to happen, smaller groups should give responsibility to the larger groups, rather than vice versa—a reasonable definition of participatory democracy.

5. The local management should be trained in appropriate 'power with' managerial styles. This approach should become embedded in the new structures. This managerial style will lead to greater local inter-active decision-making, and help to focus decisions on a human scale.

6. The local management should have a single budget that can be used for any of the health-promoting activities defined by the community. This simple organisational change would undermine much of the budget rivalry that often disrupts attempts to improve health.

7. The system should recognise that enduring public health improvements are best created when the community is involved in the decision-making process.

8. This wide remit implies that our new organisations will need to:

- be representative of the community;
- provide leadership;
- foster relationships that will allow genuine partnerships, and so manage the infrastructure in a co-operative way;
- plan for regeneration and renewal; and
- have a regulatory and public protection role.

Organisations that are moulded by these values, principles, aspirations and rules of engagement would carry out most of the activities that now fall to local government. Thus our new organisations for the promotion of health should effectively become units of local governance. The evolution of these new organisational forms will differ from place to place throughout the world. Each country and society will afford different opportunities for creative and brave people to make the necessary changes. Based on my extensive UK experience, I will illustrate the development of new health-promoting organisations by reference to the changes taking place in primary health care in the UK at the moment. The rest of this chapter will:

- describe the current situation in primary care in the UK;
- describe the government's initiatives for change in the health care system, and the philosophy underlying these;
- show how these might be built on to create structures which meet the requirements that I have outlined;
- indicate several of the health benefits we might expect from the new structures; and
- examine how these new structures could regulate themselves.

Building new organisations for health and health care: the UK as an example

The tradition of general practice in England is that around 2,000 people in a defined geographic area relate to one medically qualified practitioner, to whom they go for all their health problems. This arrangement is popular, as personal interaction between the practitioner and patient is possible, and the practitioner's awareness of the patient's problems is based on direct experience, often sustained over a long time. Repeated surveys have shown the value patients put on seeing a familiar face when they go to their practitioner. This is a marker of the importance of human scale in the pursuit of health.

Evolution of traditional general practice

Over the past 30 years, the involvement of other health professionals who contribute to the provision of good care has strengthened practices. Thus nurses, social workers, advisory officers, counsellors, alternative therapists, physiotherapists and occupational therapists have joined practice teams. Lone practitioners have increasingly found themselves unable to cope with changing medical practice and the increasing public demands on their time. It is no longer possible for these lone practitioners to look after their patients 24 hours a day, every day of the year. Thus practices have joined together to form groups, a move which has also facilitated the involvement of different categories of health workers. These group practices are usually based on one site which, in well run practices, ensures that communication between all those involved in the care of an individual is easy. So although patients do not have as intimate a relationship with their health care professionals as formerly, they have the confidence of knowing that all members of the team looking after them are able to meet and speak together with ease.

These traditional practice arrangements meet many of the requirements for human-scale health promotion and care, but judged against the core values that we wish to see in our new organisations, several essentials are missing. For instance, although general practices are called primary care teams, implying that they promote good health, most of their work is caring for people who are already ill. Therefore they should more accurately be called primary 'sickness' teams. Where practices develop a genuine health promoting role, this is usually restricted to personal health care advice. Although important, this is but a small part of the profile of public health. Moreover, the present organisation and financing of group practices makes it virtually impossible for them to be effectively involved in the wider environmental and social issues that are so important to health.

Even when treating illness, problems may arise. When patients are referred to hospitals, hospital doctors often take over responsibility for both the technology and the overall planning of care. Unfortunately the richness of a patient's story, usually best known to the general practitioner, is seldom heard in hospitals. The capacity of the patient and their local health professionals to control their care is diluted. So even when patients in hospital are involved in decisions about their care, there is likely to be an imbalance in favour of technology rather than humanity. Similarly, when patients are referred to social services, practices again lose responsibility for the provision of care. Here organisational and financial barriers frustrate local providers of care in their attempts to keep the essential human relationships intact.

Perhaps the most important defect in the present arrangements is the style of management. As has been repeatedly stressed, the 'how' and the 'where' of managers matters just as much as the 'who'. Management needs to be supportive, not oppressive, and local not distant. The management of practices is presently in the hands of the medical practitioners, closely overseen by the health authorities. The managerial style is that of the rest of the health service, and indeed the government: the rhetoric is devolution, the reality is considerable central control. There have been valiant attempts by committed health care workers to involve patients and citizens in management, and so wrest authority back to the local people, but these have usually faltered for want of wider support.

Engaging the community is essential for improving health and health care; therefore management that obstructs this objective must be changed. In our new organisations, the managerial clout of a local community working together should ensure that decisions about health are taken by, and in the interests of, local people.

Government initiatives for change in the UK health system

The UK government wishes primary care teams to be more involved in the promotion of health. They recognise that this will not be possible without change, and have initiated a number of policy developments that are potentially helpful to health as much as to health care. There is the devolution of powers to Scotland, Wales and Northern Ireland. There is the work of the Social Exclusion Unit, particularly the New Deal for Communities, which aims to reduce the inequalities between the 'haves' and the 'have-nots'. There are the health and education 'action zones' where different agencies act together to deliver benefits that will undoubtedly influence health. There are also health improvement programmes for communities to identify priorities for health. To help people's access to health care, communities are encouraged to develop drop-in clinics in supermarkets and other accessible places, and there is a telephone inquiries facility (NHS direct). Finally there are the organisational changes in the arrangements for primary care. In England these changes started with the formation of Primary Care Groups that are expected to evolve over time to Primary Care Trusts.

The philosophy underlying all these UK initiatives is threefold. The present government wishes to provide structures and incentives so that local communities can play a more active role in identifying and resolving their own problems. Where policies affect the health of individuals and communities, but are delivered by separate agencies, it wishes to break down the barriers. Finally, it wishes to ensure that people get rapid and efficient access to health care at times convenient to them, and in ways that are easily understood. These changes are quite consistent with reorienting health systems along the lines advocated in this Briefing, but to clothe the rhetoric in reality will be difficult. To develop the new structure of local governance needed to deliver this policy, politicians will need to devolve power, as well as responsibility, to an extent for which there is no precedent or blueprint—for the powerful, whilst happy to devolve responsibility, are often reluctant to devolve power. The present UK government shows no great inclination to buck this trend. It will take community leadership, courage and considerable perseverance to shift the balance of power from our present political elite to a local level. Only then can we ensure that any new clothes are tailored to the wearer's wants, not basement bargains from a government warehouse. However, when the balance of power is located at community level, we in the UK will be able to build on these government initiatives to create organisations that will transform our health and health care.

In other parts of the world, governments rarely even articulate people-friendly policies for health, and there is an even greater imbalance of power between the centre and the community. Many local communities will need to struggle vigorously to stimulate government initiatives that they can incorporate into their drive to build their healthy societies. In line with the philosophy of Lao Tze, each community will need to start the journey of change from their present position.

Creating the new health systems

*"The art of politics is to anticipate the inevitable
and facilitate its occurrence."* Talleyrand

The next section shows how a health system for the 21st century can be developed in the UK reflecting the philosophy outlined, and building on these many initiatives.

Primary Care Groups

In April 1999, general practices in England came together to form Primary Care Groups. These cover a population of around 100,000. Their board of management is clearly weighted in favour of medically trained professionals, none of whom are elected by the local community (see Box 15).

This unelected doctor-biased managerial arrangement, though not ideal, can be constructive. Doctors still enjoy the trust of local people, to a much greater extent than for example politicians or journalists.[52] Provided they act as informed advisors to a wider local panel to whom they are answerable, and so exercise leadership *with* the local community, their advocacy and leadership will be very

---

Box 15: Management Board of Primary Care Groups in the UK

- 4–7 GPs (decided by discussion among the GPs).
- 1 or 2 community or practice nurses, appointed by a selection committee.
- 1 lay member, appointed by the health authority.
- 1 social services nominee.
- 1 chief executive* appointed by the health authority.
- 1 health authority non-executive member*

The chairman is chosen from among the board members (apart from those who are ineligible*). If the GPs so wish, it has to be a GP.

helpful. In this role, doctors and other professionals on the management boards could bring relevant information and advice to forums of local people, who could then be involved in setting the agenda for any action. To be effective in a reoriented health system, professionals need to suggest solutions, not impose decisions. This role for professionals demands a community development approach to health and health care. A major part of the working in our new system should be through the community development approach.

Citizens involved in community development do not recognise the arbitrary boundaries set up for the convenience of bureaucracies. Our new organisational systems will need to control budgets relating to, for instance, housing and community facilities, and be able to make imaginative employment decisions. Viewed from a local perspective, these budgets are often separate and remote. They will need to be brought together into a single local financial pot. As this happens, local people will have increasing responsibilities, and their management board's membership will need to reflect these.

Developing local governance

As they evolve, these new organisations will embrace more and more of the functions of local government, as the local population comes to recognise that each function has implications for the public health.

Our new organisations, which started as Primary Care Groups (PCGs), will over time develop partnerships with so many formal and informal local organisations that new and effective units of local governance will emerge. Imbued with the values we suggest are relevant to our new health organisations, they will be responsible for considerable amounts of money and much of the decision-making presently made at local council, or even county and national levels. The government's primary care legislation in the UK is permissive to this evolutionary role.

This evolutionary path reflects the need to put population and individual health at the centre of local planning. The emerging organisations will draw on the many effective local initiatives that relate to health. Ultimately, those involved in the provision of education, housing, public facilities and transport will be working together within a single organisation and with a single budget. The shared values, shared budget and shared organisational structure will help to forge partnership between local citizens. This partnership will act as a network. Information will flow freely between the nodes of the network, and leadership will be located with the most appropriate people. Each decision of the management board will be taken in the interests of health, as defined by an informed and engaged local population. A network of local people with different expertise will be working in equal partnerships and in a single organisational structure. These locally constructed partnerships would promote the health of people, and of the planet, as the main goal of human societies. They would work to reverse the discontinuity that permeates and perpetuates the present arrangements. The mantra of economic growth as the sole good will be muted.

There will still be difficult decisions about capital investment for, and location of, new health care facilities. These may well need to be made by a group of local organisations working together, and structures to enable good group working will need to be developed.

Even in the best possible system dedicated to promoting good health, people will fall ill. The treatment role of doctors and other health workers in our new system will be no different from that of workers in enlightened group practices. The new role of health professionals is in advocacy and education, so that all can understand the wider health implications of local initiatives. Because of these additional functions, health workers will give leadership through advocacy and example, rather than direct involvement.

This transition of our health systems to units of local governance will take years, and the pace of change will be variable. There are a number of ways in which the evolution could be facilitated. First, to gain the confidence necessary for success, the starting point of each initiative must have well documented health benefits that the community supports. Here the role of well-trusted health care workers is crucial, as is the work that many are doing on health, or social and environmental impact assessments. They will be able to offer information about both health and health care in which the community can have confidence. They can also help to deal with the painful ethical decisions that are an inevitable part of health care delivery.

Health benefits
In the recent health publication, 'Our Healthier Nation',[53] the UK government set four priority areas in which it wishes to see health improvements, namely: heart disease and strokes; accidents; cancer; and mental health (particularly a reduction in suicide rates).

The paradox of public health is that we have known for years how to prevent these problems. To radically reduce morbidity and mortality from heart disease and strokes, the population needs to be fitter, slimmer, smoke less, feel valued and be able to contribute to their communities. Furthermore there is an important population dimension to the actions we need to take.[54] For instance, if we wish to reduce the level of alcoholism in our community, reduction of consumption by each and every person is more effective than targeting those with an alcohol problem. Likewise to prevent accidents, streets need to be safe from traffic, and homes and workplaces designed around the needs of those that live and work within them. The process of social and environmental impact assessment will help to identify what changes need to be made. Further, we know that many cancers have environmental causes.[55] Smoking, a habit predominantly enjoyed by the less materially and socially affluent, is the major cause of lung cancer. Finally, suicide is more common in people who feel that their life is pointless, who are not usefully engaged in society, and who lack social support networks.

Linking causes and solutions

As with much of our ill health, these diseases have common causes in the social and environmental circumstances of peoples' lives. So do several other problems, which our health promoting systems will need to tackle, and which are therefore added to the list. These are the need to: improve air quality; reduce fossil fuel use; and find a compassionate way to look after our elderly. There are ways of combating stroke, heart disease, accidents and suicides that at the same time improve air quality, reduce fossil fuel consumption and provide a compassionate way for looking after our elderly. Our proposed management structure, overseeing a unified budget and working in conjunction with the local community, is in a strong position to implement the necessary actions. We show below how just a few initiatives could have widely beneficial health effects.

1. Air pollution is frequently cited by local people as a major concern. The main cause is fossil fuel combustion, and any reduction in the use of fossil fuels will therefore be helpful in reducing pollution. Five ways of reducing fossil fuel use are:

- conservation of energy through home insulation;

- the generation of renewable energy;
- the creation of a community in which people have less need and desire to travel;
- walking or cycling short distances (75% of all journeys in the UK are below 5 miles, 50% below 2 miles); and
- when needed, using transport that is shared, and based on anything other than the combustion engine.

A primary care organisation could start a programme of home insulation, training and employing local people to insulate homes. Part of the payment could be in time money, which can be used within a local community to enhance social cohesion and to pay for essentials. Further, given that some 20% of houses are damp and likely to engender illness, health professionals could prescribe damp-proofing and insulation as a preventive measure. Increasing the availability and uptake of renewable energy will create job opportunities as well as improve the environment. The accompanying health benefits would motivate a local organisation to achieve these.

2. Information about health, stressing both what can and can't be done, is becoming widely available through the internet. However, to access reliable health information requires a trusted navigator, and a trusted advocate. Young people are particularly adept at using the internet, and a helpful way of involving them in the community would be as guides to this technology. Other locals could be trained to be patient advocates, working with the material generated from the net.

3. Local communities know best what their particular health problems are. A participative local community would be able to suggest areas for appropriate research, as well as being actively involved in this. Furthermore, the experiential knowledge of patients could be used in the continuing education of their health workers, as well as feeding into the education of medical and other health worker students.

4. Food quality is becoming an increasing problem. There is enormous potential for organically produced homegrown food, even in city areas. As well as encouraging local production, adjacent urban and rural areas could form partnerships to share resources. In some regions moves have been made to implement such projects (for instance farmers' markets in the UK and USA).

These measures, which produce both clear and immediate bene-fits to the community including an increase in the level of community involvement, have other helpful consequences too. The take-up of simple primary and secondary prevention measures is presently poor. Examples are the use of aspirin, stopping smoking and increasing exercise for the prevention of heart disease, stroke, colon cancer and osteoporosis. Peer group support is known to be very important in helping people take up these simple measures. A community which has networks that are achieving clear health benefits is a community that can improve the take-up of these health-enhancing activities. The recreational clubs and associations that form when communities talk and act together are important evidence of a healthy society.

To measure progress, social and environmental impact assessments at personal, household and workplace levels should be undertaken. The cost of the survey and implementing initiatives that might arise from the findings could be paid for in part by time money.

Monitoring and regulation

Citizens, patients, purchasers and providers of care will all be motivated to monitor the health changes. It would be advisable to have collectively agreed markers relevant to each intervention that can be used to measure changes. Performance then needs to be compared and publicly debated each year. Developing collectively agreed markers to measure change will not be easy, but there are sensible guidelines that could be followed.

- The markers must be relevant to the area of quality being investigated, and based on the best available evidence (incorporating the views of patients and other citizens).
- The views and concerns of the end-user should be at the heart of any appraisal.
- The information must be easy to collect, and not impose additional pressures on service providers. For this reason, there should be as few measures as possible, preferably based on information that is already collected locally.
- The information must be up-to-date and available without delay, preferably on an easily accessible website.

- At least some of the measures should be available in each locality so that accurate comparisons can be made, and localities can learn from each other.
- The measures must be easy to validate by a locally constituted group. Peer groups from adjacent localities should also be involved in monitoring progress.
- Qualitative assessments, for instance about communications and interpersonal relationships, are as important as quantitative ones. Measures should be encouraged that reflect the substance, as well as the structure, of the organisation.
- There is a plethora of information within the health service, and about the community, gathered by many other statutory organisations. However, little of it is citizen-friendly, and virtually none citizen-inspired; so in considering measures, those which are not helpful should be disposed of.

There is a considerable interest in, and action on, the development of relevant community indicators that could help guide our health structures. Information about these can be obtained from the Centre of Participation at the New Economics Foundation, and from an organisation called Redefining Progress (RP). The latter has recently produced two relevant papers: 'Lessons learned from the history of social indicators', and 'A community indicators case study—addressing the quality of life in a community'.

To put all the above into practice needs leadership. There is huge potential for improvement in the health service, and there is a significant number of people working in local communities who have the talent and energy to lead the necessary changes. My hope is that this Briefing will provide them with the appropriate facts and stimulus to help them in this task. ✾

Contacts

Citizens' Juries
Institute of Public Policy Research
30-32 Southampton Street, London WC2E 7RA.
Tel: +44 (0)20 7470 6100. <www.ippr.org.uk>

Jubilee 2000 Coalition
1 Rivington Street, London EC2A 3DT.
Tel: +44 (0)20 7739 1000. <mail@jubilee2000uk.org>
<www.jubilee2000.uk.org>

Medact
601 Holloway Rd, London N19 4DJ.
Tel: +44 (0)20 7272 2020. <www.medact.org>

New Economics Foundation
Cinnamon House, 6-8 Cole Street, London SE1 4YH.
Tel: +44 (0)20 7 407 7447. <info@neweconomics.org>
<www.neweconomics.org>

Natural Step Organisation
André Heinz, TNS International, Wallingatan 22, SE 111-24,
Stockholm, Sweden. <www.naturalstep.org>

People Centred Development Forum
<www.iisd1.iisd.ca/pcdf/>

Redefining Progress
1 Kearny Street, 4th Floor, San Francisco, CA 94108, USA.
Tel: +1 (415) 781 1191, Fax: +1 (415) 781 1198.
<info@rprogress.org> <www.rprogress.org>

SUSTAIN Alliance for Better Food and Farming
94 White Lion Street, London N1 9PF.
Tel: +44 (0)20 7 837 1228. <www.sustainweb.org>

Appendix II
References

1. *UNDP Human Development Report* (1998). Oxford University Press.
2. Lenaghan, J. (1998). *Brave New NHS: the impact of the new genetics on the health service.* Institute of Public Policy Research.
3. Bergstom, S. and Mocumbi, P. (1996). Health for all by the year 2000? *British Medical Journal*; 313: p.316.
4. As 1.
5. Marmot, M.G. *et al* (1997). Contribution of job control and other risk factors to social variations in coronary heart disease incidence. *The Lancet*; 350: pp.235-39.
6. European Environment Agency/United Nations Environment Program (1998). *Chemicals in Europe: low doses, high stakes?*
7. 1998 Aids conference, Geneva.
8. Zulma, A. & Grange, J. (1999). Doing Something about Tuberculosis. *British Medical Journal*; 318: p.956
9. Stewart Brown, S. *et al* (1997). Emotional health problems are the most important cause of disability in adults of working age: a study in the four countries of the old Oxford region. *Journal of Epidemiology and Community Health*; 51(6): pp.672-675.
10. Money, M. (1996). *Dimensions of positive mental health.* Occasional paper series by Institute for Health, Liverpool John Moores University.
11. McKeown, T. and Lowe, C.R. (1974). *An Introduction to Social Medicine.* 2nd Ed. Blackwell, Oxford.
12. Mackenbach, J.P. *et al* (1990). 'Avoidable' mortality and health services: a review of aggregate data studies, *Journal of Epidemiology and Community Health;* 44: pp.106-111.
13. Capra, F. (1983). *The Turning Point.* Flamingo, London.
14. Douthwaite, R. 'A new way to age.' *Source magazine*, Oct/Nov 1999.
15. Murray C.J. *et al* (1997). Mortality by cause for eight regions of the world: Global Burden of Disease Study. *The Lancet;* 349: pp.1269-76.
16. WHO Regional Office for Europe. *Walking and Cycling in the City.* UNDP Human Development Reports.
17. Abel Smith, B. & Townsend, P. (1965). *The poor and the poorest.* Bell, London.
18. Harrington, M. (1962). *The Other America—Poverty in the United States.* Macmillan, New York.
19. Acheson, D. (1998). *Independent inquiry into inequalities in health report.* London Stationery Office.
20. As 5.
21. Hills, John (1998). *Income and Wealth: the latest evidence.* Joseph Rowntree Foundation.
22. As 1., Chapter 1.
23. Korten, David, founder and director of the People-Centred Development Forum, (1995). *When Corporations Rule the World.* Kumarian Press, Connecticut.
24. Syme, S. *et al* (1997). 'Explaining inequalities in heart disease'. *The Lancet;* 350: p.231.

25. Putman, R.D. *et al* (1993). *Making Democracy work: Civic Traditions in Modern Italy.* Princeton University Press.
26. Various statistics from the Soil Association, SUSTAIN, and the UK Ministry for Agriculture Fisheries and Food. **Further details available from these organisations.**
27. Glynis Bath, Health Improvement Manager, Mid Devon Primary Health Group (personal communication).
28. *The Lancet* (1999); 353: pp.874-8
29. Abby *et al* (1999). *American Journal of Respiratory Critical Care Medicine;* 159: pp.373-82.
30. Jacobson, J.L. and Jacobson, S.W. (1996). Intellectual impairment in children exposed to PCBs in utero. *New England Journal of Medicine* 335: pp.783-789
31. The nine POPs that are insecticides are DDT, aldrin, dieldrin, endrin, chlordane, heptachlor, hexachlorobenzene, mirex, and toxaphone.
32. Girardet, H. (1999). *Creating Sustainable Cities.* Schumacher Briefing No 2.
33. Wilkinson, R. *et al* (1996). *Health and Social Organisation: towards a health policy for the 21st Century.* Routledge.
34. Dumfries and Galloway Health Board (1995). *Scottish Health Feedback: Patients' priorities for quality in health care.*
35. Richards, T. (1999). Patients' priorities. *British Medical Journal;* 318: p.277.
36. Claire Rayner, Chairman of the Patients' Association.
37. Reason, P. (1998). Co-operative enquiry as a discipline of professional practice. *Journal of Interprofessional Care;* 12(4): p.419.
38. Can Illness help you be a better doctor? *Hospital Doctor;* 12/8/99
39. Fisher P. & Ward A. (1994). Complementary Medicine in Europe. *British Medical Journal;* 309: pp.107-111.
40. Zollman C. & Vickers A. (1999). Complementary medicine and the patient. *British Medical Journal;* 319: pp.1558-1561.
41. As 42.
42. Barry, M. *et al* (1997). *Disease Management and Clinical Outcomes* 1: pp.5-14.
43. Macfarlane, T.J. *et al* (1997). *British Journal of General Practice;* 47: pp.719-22.
44. Salmon, P. (1999). Patients' perceptions of medical explanations for somatisisation disorders: qualitative analysis. *British Medical Journal;* 318: pp.372.
45. Montiel, R.P. and Barten, F. (1999). Urban governance and health development in Leon, Nicaragua. *Environment and Urbanisation;* 11(1).
46. Coote, A. & Lenaghan, J. *Citizens' Juries: Theory into Practice.* IPPPR.
47. Naylor, D. (1995). Grey zones of clinical practice: some limitations to evidence based medicine. *The Lancet;* 345: p.840.
48. Chalmers, I. (1998). Unbiased, relevant, and reliable assessments in health care. *British Medical Journal;* 317: p.1167.
49. Bradburn, J. *et al* (1995). Developing clinical trial protocols; the use of patient focus groups. *Psycho-Oncology;* 4: pp.107-12.
50. Nye Bevan.
51. As 23.
52. MORI Poll commissioned by the British Medical Association and reported in *Hospital Doctor* 28/1/99.
53. UK Department of Health (1999). *Saving Lives: Our Healthier Nation.* London Stationery Office.
54. Geoffrey Rose and Durkheim.
55. As 6.

SCHUMACHER BRIEFINGS

The Schumacher Society is now extending its outreach with the Schumacher Briefings—carefully researched, clearly written and well designed 20,000 word booklets on key aspects of sustainable development, to be published three times a year. They offer readers:

- background information and an overview of the issue concerned
- an understanding of the state of play in the UK and elsewhere
- best practice examples of relevance for the issue under discussion
- an overview of policy implications and implementation.

The following other Briefings have been published:

No 1: Transforming Economic Life: A Millennial Challenge
by James Robertson, published in co-operation with the New Economics Foundation. Chapters include: Transforming the System; A Common Pattern; Sharing the Value of Common Resources; Money and Finance; and The Global Economy.

No 2: Creating Sustainable Cities by Herbert Girardet. Shows how cities can dramatically reduce their consumption of resources and energy, and at the same time greatly improve the quality of life of their citizens. Chapters include: Urban Sustainability; Cities and their Ecological Footprint; The Metabolism of Cities; Prospects for Urban Farming; and Smart Cities and Urban Best Practice.

No 4: The Ecology of Money by Richard Douthwaite. This Briefing explains why money has different effects according to its origins and purposes. Was it created to make profits for a commercial bank, or issued by a government as a form of taxation, or created by its users themselves purely to facilitate their trade? And was it made in the place where it is used, or did local people have to provide goods and services to outsiders to get enough of it to trade among themselves? The Briefing shows that to build a just and sustainable world, money creation must be democratised and the payment of interest on money in circulation scrapped.

Future Briefings will deal with issues such as education, food and farming, globalisation, local development, environmental ethics, energy policy, alternatives to genetic engineering and green technology. To order a subscription, or for further details, please contact the Schumacher Society office (see over).

In the USA, Schumacher Briefings are distributed by
Chelsea Green Publishing Company of White River Junction, VT.
(800) 639-4099

THE SCHUMACHER SOCIETY
See the whole, make the connections, identify appropriate scale

The Society builds on the legacy of economist and philosopher E. F. Schumacher, author of seminal books such as *Small is Beautiful*, *Good Work* and *A Guide for the Perplexed*. Guided by his intensely practical as well as spiritually informed vision, Schumacher wanted to give societies, communities and individuals appropriate tools for change. The Schumacher Society promotes human-scale solutions for an enhanced relationship between people and the environment.

At the heart of the Society's work are the Schumacher Lectures, held in Bristol every year since 1978, and now also in Liverpool and Manchester. At the lectures, distinguished speakers from all over the world discuss key aspects of the sustainable wellbeing of people living in harmony with the earth. Speakers have included Amory Lovins, Herman Daly, Petra Kelly, Jonathon Porritt, James Lovelock, Wangari Maathai, Matthew Fox, Sir James Goldsmith, Susan George, Patrick Holden, George Monbiot, Maneka Gandhi, James Robertson and Vandana Shiva.

The main focus of the Society is educational work. Tangible expressions of our efforts over the last 20 years are: the Schumacher Lectures; Resurgence Magazine; Green Books publishing house; Schumacher College at Dartington, and the Small School at Hartland, Devon, a demonstration model of human-scale education.

The Society is based in London and Bristol. It is a non-profit making company limited by guarantee. We receive charitable donations through the Environmental Research Association based in Hartland, Devon.

Schumacher Society Members receive:

• A free lecture ticket or a cassette tape
• The Schumacher Newsletter
• Information about Schumacher College Courses and other events

The Schumacher Society, The CREATE Centre,
Smeaton Road, Bristol BS1 6XN. Phone & fax: 0117 903 1081.
<schumacher@gn.apc.org> <www.oneworld.org/schumachersoc>

A list of books of related interest is available from:

The Schumacher Book Service c/o GreenSpirit Books,
14 Beckford Close, Warminster, Wilts BA12 9LW.
Phone & Fax 01985 215679 <alan@csbooks.karoo.co.uk>
<www.greenspirit.org.uk/books>